Cooking Up Fun
for Kids with Diabetes

Patti B. Geil, MS, RD, FADA, CDE
Tami A. Ross, RD, LD, CDE

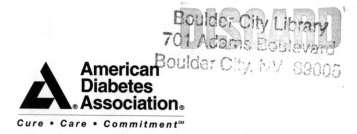

American
Diabetes
Association®

Cure • Care • Commitment℠

Director, Book Publishing, John Fedor; *Associate Director, Consumer Books,* Sherrye Landrum; *Editor,* Abe Ogden; *Associate Director, Book Production,* Peggy M. Rote; *Composition,* Circle Graphics; *Cover Design,* Koncept Inc.; *Printer,* Port City Press.

Printed in the United States of America
1 3 5 7 9 10 8 6 4 2

The suggestions and information contained in this publication are generally consistent with the *Clinical Practice Recommendations* and other policies of the American Diabetes Association, but they do not represent the policy or position of the Association or any of its boards or committees. Reasonable steps have been taken to ensure the accuracy of the information presented. However, the American Diabetes Association cannot ensure the safety or efficacy of any product or service described in this publication. Individuals are advised to consult a physician or other appropriate health care professional before undertaking any diet or exercise program or taking any medication referred to in this publication. Professionals must use and apply their own professional judgment, experience, and training and should not rely solely on the information contained in this publication before prescribing any diet, exercise, or medication. The American Diabetes Association—its officers, directors, employees, volunteers, and members—assumes no responsibility or liability for personal or other injury, loss, or damage that may result from the suggestions or information in this publication.

♾ The paper in this publication meets the requirements of the ANSI Standard Z39.48-1992 (permanence of paper).

ADA titles may be purchased for business or promotional use or for special sales. To purchase this book in large quantities, or for custom editions of this book with your logo, contact Lee Romano Sequeira, Special Sales & Promotions, at the address below, or at LRomano@diabetes.org or 703-299-2046.

American Diabetes Association
1701 North Beauregard Street
Alexandria, Virginia 22311

Library of Congress Cataloging-in-Publication Data

Geil, Patti Bazel
    Cooking up fun for kids with diabetes / Patti B. Geil, Tami A. Ross
        p. cm.
    Includes index.
    Summary: Discusses healthy eating and nutrition for children with type 1 and type 2 diabetes and provides recipes for main dishes, snacks, and desserts. Includes "fun food facts."
    ISBN 1-58040-134-1 (pbk. : alk. Paper)
        1. Diabetes in children—Diet therapy—Recipes—Juvenile literature. 2. Diabetes in children—Diet therapy—Juvenile literature. 3. Children—Nutrition—Juvenile literature. [1. Diabetics—Nutrition. 2. Diabetes. 3. Nutrition. 4. Cookery.] I. Ross, Tami. II. Title.

RJ420.D5G45 2003
641.5'6314—dc21

                                                                          2003044402

To Andrew, my tiniest taste-tester.

—T.A.R.

To Jack, Kristen, and Rachel—
Thanks for putting the fun into my cooking!

—P.B.G.

Contents

ONE

Fun in the Kitchen

Food is fun! The smell of a freshly sliced orange, the sound of popcorn popping, and the rainbow of colors on a tray of fresh vegetables can bring a smile to your face no matter how old you are. But if you have diabetes, the fun in food can quickly disappear. Instead of enjoying food, you have to treat it like medicine. You eat certain foods at certain times in certain amounts. It's all so controlled! Where's the fun in that?

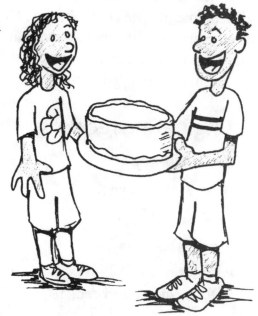

Well, food doesn't have to be so boring. You may have diabetes, but you should still enjoy what you eat. That's why we created this book. We wanted to bring fun and enjoyment back to food. We wanted kids with diabetes (and their families!) to have fun making food and have fun eating food. We hope this book helps you do both.

> *Cooking is at once child's play and adult joy. And cooking done with care, is an act of love.*
> **Chef Craig Claiborne**

There are some things about food you need to keep in mind. For example, nutrition can help you feel well and keep your diabetes under control. Enjoying food doesn't mean forgetting about what is good for you. Food is a very important part of controlling your *blood glucose*, which plays a big part in how well you feel. How can you have fun if your blood glucose is too low and you feel dizzy and shaky? How can you enjoy eating if your blood glucose is too high and you feel tired and worn out? The first ingredient to fun in the kitchen is feeling good. So before we talk about anything else, let's talk about eating healthy (don't worry, we'll keep it short).

Healthy Eating Is Fun! (Believe It or Not)

Okay, so you probably think the words "healthy" and "delicious" don't belong in the same sentence. You may think foods that are good for you will automatically taste bad. Just because a food is good for you doesn't mean it has to be boring. Healthy food can be fun and actually pretty tasty. In this book, we've put together some recipes that are not only a blast to make and eat, but they're good for you too.

But what does "good for you" mean? It can mean lots of things, such as low in fat, or high in vitamins, or low in carbohydrate, or even just small portions. A healthy, balanced diet, low in fat and sweets, is good for all kids whether they have type 1 diabetes or type 2 diabetes—or no diabetes at all! So, before we start talking about fats and carbohydrates and all of that other stuff, let's talk about healthy eating for type 1 and type 2.

Fun food fact!

Americans eat more than three and a half million tons of cheese a year. That's enough cheese to build a cheese wall six feet high and one foot thick around the state of Texas.

Original kid recipe

Baked Turkey

FROM: **Maggie, age 6**

PREP TIME: **2 hours**

NUMBER OF SERVINGS: **5**

INSTRUCTIONS:
Catch a turkey and cook it.

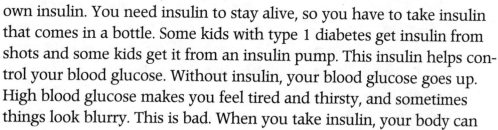

For Kids with Type 1 Diabetes

If you have type 1 diabetes, it means that your body can't make its own insulin. You need insulin to stay alive, so you have to take insulin that comes in a bottle. Some kids with type 1 diabetes get insulin from shots and some kids get it from an insulin pump. This insulin helps control your blood glucose. Without insulin, your blood glucose goes up. High blood glucose makes you feel tired and thirsty, and sometimes things look blurry. This is bad. When you take insulin, your body can use the blood glucose and your blood glucose will go lower. But if you take too much insulin, your blood glucose can go too low and you can feel shaky and dizzy. This is very bad. If your blood glucose goes *really* low, you can pass out. This is very, very bad. If you take just the right amount, your blood glucose will be on target and you'll feel great!

In the 15th century, when Dutch pirates found a load of chocolate on a ship they had raided, they threw it overboard in disgust. The Spanish and Portuguese had kept chocolate a secret from the rest of Europe. The pirates didn't know they were throwing away a delicious treat from the Americas!

So what makes your blood glucose rise in the first place? One thing is food. When you eat (or drink) something that contains carbohydrate, your body turns it into blood glucose. If you eat lots of carbohydrate, your blood glucose will go very high. If you eat a small amount of carbohydrate, your blood glucose will only rise a little bit. You probably can't take the same amount of insulin every time you eat. If you took the same amount of insulin for a small snack as you did for an all-you-can-eat buffet, your blood glucose would go very low!

The trick is to match up the amount of insulin you take to the amount of food you eat. Since every kid is different, we can't tell you how much insulin you should take, or how much food to eat. Your doctor, registered dietitian (a nutrition expert), and parents will help you do that. What you need to know is this—how much food you eat is very important.

It sounds crazy, but you are actually very lucky. Doctors have learned a lot about diabetes over the years and it is treated very differently than it used to be. People with diabetes used to have to eat special diets. Back in the old days, they had to boil their food and eat things like limewater with bread and butter, or plain blood pudding. Talk about yucky! And they couldn't eat anything sweet at all! In fact, the diet for diabetes was so bad that people used to call it "rabbit food."

Today, we understand a lot more about diabetes. Now we know that you can eat the same foods as other kids. You probably shouldn't eat a lot of sweets, and regular soda with sugar probably isn't a good idea either. But all kids should stay away from a lot of sweets and soda! Your registered dietitian will help you and your parents figure out what foods are good for you. This doctor will come up with a meal plan that is tasty and healthy. A lot of the recipes in this book will probably work well with this meal plan. So don't worry. Just because food is good for you, does not mean it will taste yucky!

Original kid recipe

Angel Food Cake

FROM: **Steven, age 9**

PREP TIME: **0**
NUMBER OF SERVINGS: **31**

INSTRUCTIONS:
Go to the store. Buy a cake. Cut and eat.

For Kids with Type 2 Diabetes

Type 2 diabetes used to be called *adult onset diabetes*. That meant that it was something that happened mostly to adults. This is not true anymore. More and more kids have type 2 diabetes, and the number is rising quickly. Why? It has to do with what causes type 2 diabetes.

Type 2 diabetes is different than type 1 diabetes. Type 1 diabetes means that your body does not make insulin. Type 2 diabetes means your body makes insulin, it just does not make enough or it does not use the insulin very well. This is why you probably do not have to take insulin like kids with type 1 diabetes do. Doctors and scientists believe that type 2 diabetes is caused by two main things:

1. Not getting enough exercise
2. Eating too much food, which causes you to be overweight

Squirrel pie?!

The following foods were popular in America when the Declaration of Independence was signed in 1776:

Opossum stew
Pickled passenger pigeons
Milkweed shoots
Squirrel pie
Pigs' feet
Soup with marigold petals
Raspberry leaf tea
Dandelion salad

Yuck.

Thirty years ago, kids got a lot more exercise. Video games had not been invented yet, nobody owned a computer, and TV was not as good (they only had 3 channels!). To have fun, kids played outside. They rode bikes and played sports. They explored the woods behind their house or made up games. They were never sitting down for long. Kids also ate healthier food. Fast food was not as popular or as common as it is today, and the amount of food kids ate at breakfast, lunch, and dinner was smaller. They didn't have super-sized combos!

All of this meant that kids were in better shape than they are today. When you are in good shape, you usually do not get type 2 diabetes. This is why type 2 diabetes used to be called an adult disorder. Adults were out of shape. Adults did not exercise. Adults did not watch what they ate. So, adults were the ones with type 2 diabetes. Today, a lot of kids are out of shape, so a lot of kids are getting type 2 diabetes, too.

So what can you do? Like we said before, kids with type 1 diabetes take

Another word of advice

"Never tell your mom her diet's not working."

Michael, age 14

Original kid recipe

Cheese and Macaroni

FROM: **Courtney, age 10**

PREP TIME: **10 Hours**
NUMBER OF SERVINGS: **2**

INSTRUCTIONS:
Boil some water. When water is boiling, put macaroni in. When macaroni is done, put the cheese in it. Now it is time to CHOW DOWN!

Seal of approval

One day, a mother returned from the grocery store with her small son. As soon as she sat the sacks down in the kitchen, the boy pulled out a box of animal crackers he had begged for. He opened the box and spread the animal-shaped crackers all over the kitchen counter. "What are you doing?" his surprised mom asked. "The box says you can't eat them if the seal is broken," the boy explained. "I'm looking for the seal."

insulin to stay healthy. What medicine do kids with type 2 diabetes take? The answer—none at all. There is a pill that can help kids with type 2 (it's called metformin [Glucophage]),

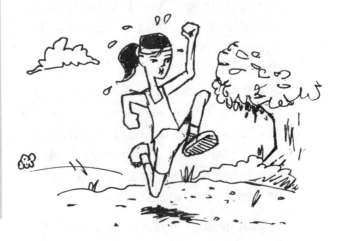

but it does not always work. Plus, it doesn't get to the root of the problem. The best "medicine" for type 2 diabetes is regular exercise and healthy eating. By getting at least 30 minutes of activity a day and cutting down on high-fat and high-calorie foods, you can help keep your type 2 diabetes under control. This is very little work when you think about how much good it can do. And you can get your family to help. If you have type 2 diabetes, your mom or dad probably has type 2 diabetes, too. Eating better and exercising is good for all of you, so get the whole family involved!

Keep an Eye Out for These Guys

Just about everything in food can affect your health in one way or another. But there are a few things you really need to watch. The following items pack the biggest wallop when it comes to your health, so stay on the lookout and be prepared.

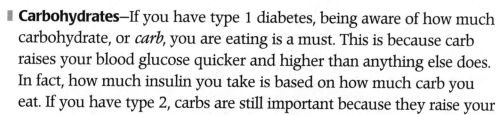

■ **Carbohydrates**—If you have type 1 diabetes, being aware of how much carbohydrate, or *carb*, you are eating is a must. This is because carb raises your blood glucose quicker and higher than anything else does. In fact, how much insulin you take is based on how much carb you eat. If you have type 2, carbs are still important because they raise your blood glucose, too. A registered dietitian can tell you and your parents more about carbs and how they come into play with your diabetes.

■ **Fat**—Foods that have a lot of fat also have a lot of calories. If you have type 2 diabetes, you probably need to eat less calories to control your weight. Staying away from foods that are high in fat is a good way to lower how many calories you eat. And since it is good for your heart, a low fat diet is good for nearly everyone.

Now that is super-sized

The following are the largest foods on record. Imagine the grams of carbohydrate!

Cookie: 81 feet, 8 inches in diameter, New Zealand, 1996

Lollipop: 1.35 tons, Denmark, 1994

Pancake: 49 feet, 3 inches in diameter, weighing 2.95 tons, England, 1994

Pizza: 122 feet, 8 inches in diameter, South Africa, 1990

Pumpkin: 1131 pounds, Altoona, PA, 1999

Sausage: 28.77 miles long, Canada, 1995

Taco: 15 feet long, 29 inches wide, weighing 747 pounds. Contained 559 pounds of meat, 46 pounds of tomatoes, 37 pounds of onions, and 18 pounds of cilantro, Texas, 1999

Sweets—These used to be strictly off-limits for people with diabetes. Now we know that sweets are just another type of carbohydrate. What does that mean? It means you can eat candy every once in awhile so long as you count it as part of your total daily carbohydrate (your parents and a dietitian can explain). But be careful—sweets can raise your blood glucose very quickly. And they are *empty calories*, which means they do not contain anything healthy like vitamins and minerals. So sweets are okay, just in small amounts.

Are you confused yet? We hope not. All of this nutrition stuff can get pretty complicated (and boring), but it is stuff every kid with diabetes needs to know. To make things easier, we wrote this book, which is filled with delicious recipes that are good for you. If you are not sure what to eat, pick something from here! All of these recipes can help you watch your weight and keep your diabetes under control. So stop reading, get cooking, and start having fun!

Why, Duke Winterbottom, you're getting capon on your marrowbone!

In medieval times, the amount of food served at royal feasts was just incredible. This is a shopping list for food served at a feast in 1387. Not a single vegetable!

1 oxen, lying in salt	50 capons (fancy word for rooster) of high grease	12 dozen young hens to roast
2 oxen, fresh		100 dozen pigeons
120 heads of sheep, fresh	8 dozen other capons	12 dozen partridges (not in a pear tree)
120 carcasses of sheep, fresh	60 dozen hens	
	200 pair rabbits	8 dozen young rabbits
12 boars	4 pheasants	12 cranes (still another type of bird)
14 calves	5 herons and bitterns (types of birds)	
140 piglets		Wild fowl (wild birds)
300 marrowbones	10 dozen curlews (another type of bird)	120 gallons milk
Lard and grease		12 gallons cream
3 tons salt venison	12 dozen wimbrels (yet another type of bird)	40 gallons curds
3 does (a female deer) fresh venison		3 bushels apples
	6 young goats	11,000 eggs
50 swans	5 dozen young hens for jelly	
210 geese		

TWO
....

Just for Grownups

You Know, the Boring Stuff

ooking with kids offers countless benefits to a family. Although the finished product is easily the most delicious result, the process of working together to create the perfect vegetable soup or banana bread can be even more important. Many of us have special memories of time spent with a parent or grandparent making a simple meal, memorable dessert, or just a floury mess in the kitchen!

In addition to the basics of meal preparation, involving kids in the kitchen teaches them a variety of important skills. Cooking requires organizational abilities from the start. Mixing and measuring develops hand-eye coordination and motor skills. Following a recipe requires reading for comprehension, as well as learning new terms such as marinate, mince, and mix. Math skills are strengthened with measuring, counting, and the multiplication needed to double or triple a recipe. Add to this the social and emotional bonuses of teamwork, communication, and self-confidence and you'll see that every moment invested in the kitchen with your child pays major dividends.

For a child with diabetes, cooking offers even more. It's an opportunity to informally learn about good nutrition. Although the task may be to prepare a simple snack, in the process kids become more familiar with different food groups and their effects on blood glucose. Picky eaters often eat better when they've been involved in the purchasing and preparation of their food—they take pride in their work! Time spent together in the kitchen lays the foundation for a healthy relationship with food.

In the last section, we covered some very rudimentary basics about nutrition. It's not really in the scope of this book to offer in-depth advice about meal planning and healthy eating—that's for you to discuss with your child's doctor and registered dietitian (RD). But the more you know, the more your child can know, which better prepares both of you for the road ahead. So in the next few pages, we'll discuss some of the foundations of healthy eating for a child with diabetes.

Which Meal Plan Is the Best?

A meal plan gives guidelines for the types and amounts of food a child with diabetes should eat at each meal and snack. No one single meal planning approach works for all children with diabetes. As the nutrition expert on the diabetes care team, the RD is a valuable guide to help you create a meal plan that is individualized to meet the special needs of your child with diabetes. Many children with diabetes use either the diabetes food pyramid, exchange list, or carbohydrate counting meal-planning approach. Following is a brief description of each.

The Diabetes Food Pyramid

The Diabetes Food Pyramid* is based on the Food Guide Pyramid developed by the US Department of Agriculture (USDA) and is described in a pamphlet available from the American Diabetes Association called *The First Step in Diabetes Meal Planning*

---

*The Food Guide Pyramid developed by the USDA is currently undergoing review and possible revision. Any changes made to the Food Guide Pyramid will possibly be reflected in a revised Diabetes Food Pyramid. For now, the current Diabetes Food Pyramid, based on the USDA model, remains the standard.

(call 1-800-DIABETES or visit *www.diabetes.org* to order a copy for your family). The diabetes pyramid has six sections, or food groups:

▮ grains, beans, and starchy vegetables   ▮ milk
▮ vegetables   ▮ meat and others
▮ fruit   ▮ fats, sweets, and alcohol

Children with diabetes should eat a variety of foods from each of the food groups every day, with grains, beans, and starchy vegetables serving as the basis of their meal plan. An RD can individualize the Diabetes Food Pyramid for your child, reevaluating the number of servings needed from each food group, keeping in mind that foods in the meat and fat group generally have less carbohydrate to affect blood glucose.

Exchange Lists

The exchange lists organize food into eight different exchange groups:

▮ bread/starch   ▮ milk   ▮ meat/protein   ▮ other carbohydrate
▮ fruit   ▮ vegetable   ▮ fat   ▮ free foods

Each serving or exchange within a group has essentially the same nutritional value, so foods in each specific exchange list can be substituted or "exchanged" with other foods from the same list. For example, you can exchange 17 small grapes for 1/2 cup of unsweetened orange juice. Or 1 slice of white bread for 3/4 cup dry cereal. An RD can work with your child to prescribe the number and type of exchanges to be eaten at each meal and snack. The exchange list meal planning approach allows consistent food and carbohydrate intake, with a wide variety of food choices.

Carbohydrate Counting

The carbohydrate counting approach has become one of the most popular for children with diabetes. With carbohydrate counting, you and your child learn about the specific amount of carbohydrate in foods, keeping in mind that carbohydrate is the nutrient that has the biggest impact on blood glucose. An RD can help you select a goal amount of carbohydrate for your child to eat at each meal and snack. The carbohydrate can be recorded as exact number of grams or as carbohydrate choices, with 15 grams of carbohydrate equaling one carbohydrate choice. Frequent blood glucose monitoring will confirm that the suggested carbohydrate intake is keeping blood glucose levels within the target range you, your doctor, and the RD agree upon. Information about the carbohydrate content of foods is available from food labels, exchange lists, or reference books.

One reason carbohydrate counting is so popular is because it allows quite a bit of flexibility in meal planning, while keeping carbohydrate intake consistent from day to day. It works especially well in children with type 1 diabetes, who can eventually learn to do advanced carbohydrate counting. Advanced carbohydrate counting involves calculating a personal insulin-to-carbohydrate ratio to determine the amount of fast-acting insulin to take prior to eating a meal or snack. The insulin dosage is based on the amount of carbohydrate in that meal. A common insulin-to-carbohydrate starting point is 1 unit of fast-acting insulin for each 15 grams of carbohydrate.

Carbohydrate counting also works well for children with type 2 diabetes. When combined with a low-fat diet and physical activity, consistent carbohydrate intake and controlled portion sizes will allow for weight loss and improved blood glucose levels.

FAQs About Food

As a parent of a child with diabetes, you probably find you have a lot more questions about diabetes care than you do answers. This is completely understandable because you care very much about the well-being of your child. Following are some of the more common questions parents have about healthy eating and how it relates to their child with diabetes.

Q *Our child has always been a picky eater. Now that he's been diagnosed with type 1 diabetes, how can we be sure he'll get enough to eat and avoid mealtime hassles?*

Nothing provokes more anxiety in a parent than a child who doesn't want to eat—except a child with diabetes who refuses to eat after receiving his mealtime dose of insulin! Poor eating habits and the potential for hypoglycemia (low blood sugar) can make mealtime a battleground, stretching the nerves of both parent and child.

▌ Start by adopting a positive attitude at meal and snack time. The foods a child with diabetes needs are the same foods that are good for the entire family, so it's best to serve one meal for everyone. This way the child with diabetes isn't signaled out as different. Your job as a parent is to put the proper food choices on the table; the job of the child with diabetes is to be responsible for what and how much to eat. Offer a healthy meal, and then relax. If you are a good role model for eating well, your child is likely to follow your lead.

▌ Although you want to avoid becoming a short-order cook, it makes sense to have two or three "second choice" foods as backups for those times when it's just not worth the fight. These foods should be easy to fix, tried and true favorites, such as a grilled cheese sandwich or peanut butter and crackers. Offer them quickly and without comment if necessary; then move on to a pleasant discussion of the day's activities.

▌ Involving your child in menu planning, food shopping, and preparing fun recipes (such as those in this book) will go a long way toward encouraging him to eat well. If it's something he's planned or prepared, chances are he'll be much more likely to gobble it up!

▌ When your child is eating well, don't forget to tell him that you're proud of him. Positive reinforcement works wonders.

One alternative may be to give your child his rapid-acting mealtime insulin after he eats, rather than before. This allows you to base his insulin dose on the amount of carbohydrate he actually ate, lowering the risk for hypoglycemia. Check with your diabetes care team for guidance.

Q *What do we do about eating for special occasions? Food has always been an important part of our holidays and celebrations. We also eat at a fast food restaurant every Friday evening as part of our weekly family night.*

Your child with diabetes certainly needs to continue to participate in family celebrations. Because food often plays a major part in special occasions, it may be necessary to make some changes in the timing or dose of insulin to keep your child's blood glucose under control after a heavy holiday meal. Another approach is to encourage physical activity. A family walk or game of basketball in the backyard will help bring blood glucose levels down after a special occasion meal.

Americans love to eat out and families with diabetes often find themselves facing high-fat/high-carbohydrate choices when they read the menu at a fast food restaurant. However, it is possible to make good choices at fast food chains. Try some of these fast food tips:

- Fast food restaurants often provide the nutrition and exchange information about their products locally or on a web site. Review this information at home so you'll be ready to order on your next outing.
- If you find yourself in a burger restaurant, encourage your child to have a *small* burger and french fries.
- Try substituting a salad with low-fat dressing for the fries every once in awhile.
- Skip the super-sizing unless your child has had or plans to have a particularly active day.
- Low-fat milk is often available as an alternative to soft drinks or shakes.
- Chicken can be a good option. Smart chicken choices are grilled or broiled, although chicken nuggets will always be popular with kids

and their carbohydrate content is not too high. Try to avoid "crispy" chicken sandwiches—these are usually loaded with fat, calories, and carb.

▌ Pizza is actually one of the healthier fast foods. It contains foods from almost all the food groups: bread, meat, vegetable, and milk. Encourage your child to top his pizza with vegetable toppings and add a salad with low-fat dressing on the side to round out the meal.

Q *My daughter loves sweets. Is sugar totally off-limits in the meal plan to control her type 2 diabetes?*

Sweets are no longer forbidden foods for children with diabetes. We know the most important factor influencing blood glucose is the *total* carbohydrate intake, rather than the *source* of the carbohydrate. Sweets should be substituted for other carbohydrate-containing foods in the meal plan, such as those in the bread or fruit groups. As with children who don't have diabetes, it's important to keep overall healthy eating goals in mind and limit sweets with empty calories. Check blood glucose levels before and about 2 hours after sweet treats to see the effect they have on your child's diabetes control.

Q *Our son is a sports fanatic. What should we do to prevent and treat hypoglycemia that may occur during practice and game situations?*

Encourage your son to stay physically active and make it easy for him to play safely and at peak performance by planning ahead for sporting events.

▌ Before your child signs up to participate in any sport, talk with your diabetes care team to adjust his individual treatment plan, if necessary. Talk to the team coach and make sure that he and your child's teammates can recognize the signs and symptoms of hypoglycemia and know what to do if it occurs. A medical identification tag is an important part of the team uniform for your child with diabetes.

▌ Extra blood glucose checks are a good idea for all athletes with diabetes. Checking blood glucose before a game or practice can help you decide whether your child needs a carbohydrate snack at the start. You may find you need to reduce the dose of insulin acting during the time of physical activity to prevent hypoglycemia. Check blood glucose about every 30 minutes during a game or practice and whenever he feels low. Head off hypoglycemia by giving him carbohydrate before his blood glucose level drops below 70 mg/dl. Low blood glucose levels can occur up to 24 hours after a game or practice as his body replaces the stored glucose he's used during strenuous exercise, so continue to check, particularly at bedtime and in the middle of the night.

▌ Carbohydrate is the body's preferred fuel during physical activity. You can supply the needed carbohydrate in the form of beverages such as sports drinks or diluted fruit juice or with carbohydrate-containing foods such as crackers, dry unsweetened cereal, fruit, popcorn, pretzels, or trail mix.

▌ Be aware of your child's symptoms of hypoglycemia, such as shakiness, sweatiness, irritability, or headache. Low blood sugar is associated with fatigue and poor athletic performance, and can lead to more severe consequences if left untreated. If your child's blood glucose level dips below 70 mg/dl, he should raise it by consuming 15 grams of carbohydrate, such as 1/2 cup undiluted fruit juice, 1/2 can regular soda, one dose of glucose gel, or 3–4 glucose tablets. If his level is still too low after 15 minutes, he should have another treatment. Follow up with an additional snack if his next meal is more than an hour away. Your son should get back in the game only after his symptoms of hypoglycemia are gone and his blood glucose has returned to his target range.

Q *Our diabetes care team has suggested that our daughter eat three meals with snacks each day. What are some healthy snack ideas?*

Whether they have diabetes or not, children's small stomachs and high activity levels mean they require frequent refueling to meet energy demands. Snacks help smooth out blood glucose control by preventing the low blood glucose levels that can occur if there is not enough food in your daughter's system. They can also curb excessive hunger, which can lead to overly large meals and subsequent high blood glucose levels. Your daughter's daily schedule and medication dose will determine her ideal snack pattern, but most families find their child with diabetes needs to eat a small snack halfway between each meal. A good snack should satisfy hunger and provide long-term appetite control. Favorite snack ideas include cheese and crackers, a meat or peanut butter sandwich, or cereal and milk. The RD on your diabetes care team can individualize a snack plan for your daughter with a target amount of carbohydrate to aim for at each meal and snack. Ideas for kid-friendly snacks with 15 grams of carbohydrate per serving include:

- 8 animal crackers
- 9–13 potato chips
- 3 cheese/peanut butter cracker sandwiches
- 3/4 cup dry unsweetened cereal
- Fruit–1/2 cup canned fruit cocktail, 1/2 cup unsweetened applesauce, or 1 small fresh fruit
- 3 graham cracker squares
- 3/4 ounce pretzels
- 24 oyster crackers
- 2/3 cup fat-free artificially-sweetened plain or fruit-flavored yogurt

Get Started Already

By now, we hope we've answered some of the questions you may have had, or at least have given you somewhere to start. So now it's time to start cooking. In the beginning, you will be tempted to make things easy on yourself—and your kitchen—by doing most of the work! After all, it is faster and less messy to do it yourself. Resist the temptation. Encourage your child with diabetes to stretch his horizons. Expect a mess, clean as you go, and keep your sense of humor close at hand. Use the recipes in this book to start simple and have fun!

How Much Help Can You Really Expect?

Although your child may be eager to dive into dinner preparation, she will still require close supervision in the kitchen. Use the following guidelines to determine safe and suitable tasks for your child.

Most 2-Year-Olds Can:	Most 3- to 5-Year-Olds Also Can:	Most 5- to 7-Year-Olds Also Can:	Most 7- to 10-Year-Olds Also Can:	Most Older Children Also Can:
Wipe table tops	Shape dough	Fill and level measuring cups and spoons	Cut with a table knife	Take the lead on menu planning and grocery shopping lists
Break apart raw cauliflower or broccoli	Add and stir cool ingredients in a bowl	Beat ingredients with a wire whisk	Use a can opener	Make recipes with multiple ingredients
Tear and wash salad greens	Scrub and wash fruits and vegetables	Spread soft spreads such as peanut butter or cream cheese	Use a microwave oven (with adult supervision)	Use a sharp knife to slice or chop (with adult supervision)
Bring ingredients to you	Pour liquids from a small pitcher	Crack an egg	Prepare simple recipes with a few ingredients	Bake or broil using the oven
	Peel oranges and hard-cooked eggs	Set timers	Grate cheese	Load the dishwasher and clean kitchen counters
	Mash bananas with a fork		Add to and stir hot mixtures	
	Set the table		Blend foods in a blender	
			Broil in a toaster oven (with adult supervision)	
			Clear and wipe the table after dinner	

Three

Kitchen Smarts for Kids Who Cook

Helpful tips that make cooking
easier, safer, and a lot more fun!

Safety First

Although time spent in the kitchen can be child's play, sharp knives and scalding water make safety a big concern. Always keep these safety tips in mind.

- An adult should always supervise when you are:
  - using the stove, oven, or microwave
  - handling hot pans, pots and bowls
  - using electrical appliances such as can openers
  - cutting or slicing food with knives

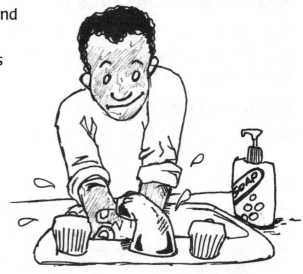

- Wash your hands with soap and hot water before you start cooking and wash them after you handle foods, especially raw eggs and meats.

Safety First (Continued)

- Never plug or unplug electrical appliances with wet hands.

- Tie back long hair, roll up loose sleeves, and cover clothes with an apron.

- Have clean, dry oven mitts and hot pads handy near the stove, oven, or microwave so you can safely handle hot pans, pots, bowls, and oven doors.

- When you cook on the stovetop, point pot handles toward the back of the stove to prevent spills.

- Clean up spills on the floor right away so you don't slip.

- Make sure the stove burners and/or oven is turned off as soon as you finish cooking.

- Be prepared for emergencies by keeping a first aid kit and fire extinguisher handy.

- Keep emergency numbers near the telephone.

Kids' Kitchen Dictionary

Young chefs need to know what they are talking about! You can build your vocabulary by getting to know the following cooking terms and techniques.

Bake: cook in the oven

Beat: make a smooth mixture by stirring strongly with a fork, spoon, whisk, or electric mixer

Blend: stir 2 or more ingredients together

Boil: cook a liquid over high heat until liquid is hot and bubbles rise to the top

Broil: cook under the broiler, or top heating element in the oven

Chill: put in the refrigerator to keep cold

Chop: cut into small pieces with a sharp knife

Coat: cover or roll food in another ingredient

Cube: cut into evenly-sized squares

Dash: one quick shake or sprinkle

Dice: cut into very small (1/4-inch) squares

Drain: pour off liquid or fat

Fold: mix gently with a rubber scraper or spoon by lifting the bottom of the mixture outwards and over the top until blended

Fry: cook in an open skillet

Garnish: decorate food with colorful additions such as parsley or slices of lemon and lime

Grate: rub food against a grater to make very small bits

Grill: broil under high heat or over hot coals

Knead: work dough by pressing and folding it with your hands

Marinate: let food soak in a flavorful liquid

Melt: heat on a stovetop or in a microwave slowly on low heat until it becomes a liquid

Mince: chop into tiny pieces

Mix: stir 2 or more ingredients together

Pare: cut off the outside skin of a food, such as carrots or cucumbers, using a peeler or a paring knife

Peel: pull off the outer skin as in peeling an orange or banana

Pinch: a small amount of seasoning that can be held between the thumb and forefinger

Puree: process or grind food into a smooth pulp in a food processor or blender

Sauté: cook in a skillet over medium to high heat while stirring constantly (also known as "stir-fry")

Season: flavor foods by sprinkling them with herbs and spices

Shred: cut into very thin strips

Simmer: cook a liquid mixture over low heat until it barely bubbles, but doesn't boil heavily

Stir: mix with a spoon in a circular motion

Toss: mix lightly and gently using salad tongs or two spoons

Whip: beat with an eggbeater or electric mixer

Whisk: beat or stir food with a wire whisk

Kitchen math

1 tablespoon = 3 teaspoons or 1/2 fluid ounce

1/2 cup = 8 tablespoons or 4 fluid ounces

1 cup = 16 tablespoons or 8 fluid ounces

1 pint = 2 cups or 16 fluid ounces

1 quart = 4 cups or 32 fluid ounces or 2 pints

1 gallon = 4 quarts or 128 fluid ounces or 8 pints

1 pound = 16 ounces

Equipment List

Following is a list of the items you will need for the recipes in this book. Look at the equipment list on each recipe to see what equipment you will need for that recipe.

Utensils

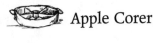 Apple Corer

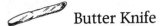 Butter Knife

Can Opener

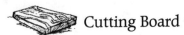 Cutting Board

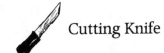 Cutting Knife

Fork

Garlic Press

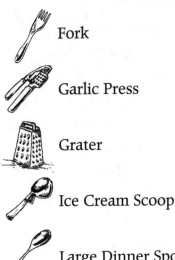 Grater

Ice Cream Scoop

Large Dinner Spoon

Long Handled
Mixing Spoon
(like a Wooden Spoon)

 Melon Scoop

 Paring Knife

 Pastry Brush

 Peeler (like a Potato
Peeler)

 Potato Masher

 Potholders

 Regular Dinner Spoon

 Small and Large
Round Cookie Cutter
(or Biscuit Cutter)

 Spatula (Metal)

Spatula (Rubber)

Whisk

 Wooden Toothpick

Measuring Utensils

 Glass Measuring Cup
(with a handle and
pouring spout; usually
holds about 2 cups)

 Measuring Cups (Set)

 Measuring Spoons
(Set)

Pots, Pans, Bowls, Etc.

 8″ X 8″ Baking Pan

 9″ X 13″ Baking Pan

 Airtight Container
(such as Tupperware)

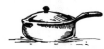 Deep Pan

 Fondue Pot or Small
Crock Pot

 Frying Pan/Skillet

Pots, Pans, Bowls, Etc. (*Continued*)

 Griddle

 Ice Cube Trays

 Large Mixing Bowl

 Loaf Pan

 Microwave-Safe Serving Dish (such as a Deep-Dish Glass Pie Plate)

 Muffin Tin (Small and Large)

 Omelet Pan

 Pitcher

 Plate

 Regular Pan

 Sauce Pan

 Serving Bowl

 Serving Dish

 Sieve

 Small Mixing Bowl

 Stockpot

 Strainer/Colander

 Wire Rack

Appliances

 Blender

 Electric Mixer

 Food Processor

 Microwave Oven

 Oven

Refrigerator

 Microwave-Safe Plastic Wrap

 Toaster

 Paper Baking Cups

 Toaster Oven

 Paper Towels

Extra Materials

 Wax-Coated Paper Cups

 Aluminum Foil

 Wooden Popsicle Sticks

 Bamboo Skewers

 Zip-Top Bag (such as Zip-Loc)

 Latex Gloves

Measuring up

Successful cooking depends on accurate measuring. Always use special measuring cups and spoons, rather than those you use for eating.

To measure liquids: use a glass or clear plastic measuring cup. Place the cup on the countertop. You may need to bend down to look at the liquid at eye level as you pour.

To measure dry ingredients: choose the proper size measuring cup or spoon. Fill to overflowing. Level by scraping across the top of the cup or spoon with the straight edge of a knife. Careful—don't pack down the ingredients unless the recipe calls for it.

Brown sugar or shortening: these ingredients call for packing into the measuring cup so there won't be any air left in the cup or spoon. Fill the right size cup with brown sugar or shortening. Push down hard with the spoon. Level off the top with the straight edge of a knife.

Four

About the Recipes

In *Cooking Up Fun for Kids with Diabetes*, we tried to base the recipes on foods that kids love. And we hope you'll agree. While you'll find old favorites, we also tried to fit in less familiar foods, such as *jicama* and *Ugli fruit* that even the pickiest eater will enjoy. The basics of healthy eating for kids with diabetes have not been forgotten either. Complete nutrient information, conducted by a third party nutrition analyst, is provided for each recipe. If you want to know how much carbohydrate you (or your child) is eating, the information is at your fingertips! Diabetes food exchange information is listed as well. You may be surprised to see that several of the recipes contain sugar, which used to be strictly off-limits for kids with diabetes. Now we know that sugars can be treated just like any other form of carbohydrate and can be eaten as long as the total amount of carbohydrate doesn't go over the planned amount for that meal or snack.

Since this book is mostly for kids, the recipes have been divided into simple steps. Getting adults involved is the best way to have the most fun—and it is required in a very few of the more complicated projects. A special "little hands" icon tells you how hard each recipe will be:

 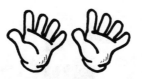 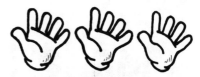

**Simple
to make**

**A bit more
challenging**

**May require the help
of an experienced cook**

There's also a flame icon that tells you if the recipe needs heat:

**A flame icon means
the recipe needs heat**

**A crossed-out flame icon means
it does not need heat**

Get ready to put the fun back into your food. Jump into these quick-to-fix, tasty, and healthy recipes and enjoy the many benefits of spending quality time with kids in the kitchen!

Made for a Meal

Main dishes, side dishes,
and appetizers that are perfect
for breakfast, lunch, or dinner

Toasted Cheese People

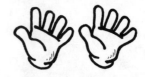

A is for American cheese.

INGREDIENTS

2 slices whole-wheat bread

1 1/2 (3/4 ounce) slices fat-free American cheese

1/4 teaspoon bacon bits

4 carrot sticks (2 inches long)

4 celery sticks (2 inches long)

EQUIPMENT

Measuring spoons

Cutting board

Knife

Small (1 3/4-inch) biscuit or cookie cutter

Large (2 1/2-inch) biscuit or cookie cutter

Baking pan

Spatula

Potholder

DO THIS FIRST

▌ Check with an adult before you begin cooking and ask for help with cutting and at the oven or toaster.

▌ Read through the whole recipe and make sure you have all of the ingredients and equipment you need.

▌ Cut carrot and celery sticks.

DIRECTIONS

1 Using a small round cookie or biscuit cutter and a large round cookie or biscuit cutter, cut a small and large circle out of each slice of whole wheat bread to make 2 heads and 2 bodies.

2 Place the bread circles on a baking pan or toaster oven pan.

3 Break off pieces of cheese and place them on the bread circles, covering the bread with cheese.

4 Use bacon bits to make eyes, a nose, and a mouth on each head and to make buttons on each body.

5 Toast in a toaster oven, or broil in an oven 4 inches from the heating element, until the cheese is melted (about 2–3 minutes). Watch closely and remove from the oven if the cheese begins to darken.

6 Using a metal spatula, carefully move the toasted cheese-bread to a plate, placing the bodies below the heads. Add carrot sticks for arms and celery sticks for legs.

PREPARATION TIME
10 minutes

BAKING TIME
2–3 minutes

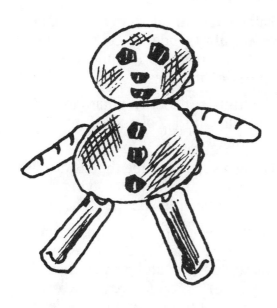

You will need a small round cookie or biscuit cutter about 1 3/4 inches wide and a large round cookie or biscuit cutter about 2 1/2 inches wide for this recipe. If you don't have the cutters, try using a clean soup can and a clean 6-ounce tomato paste can for cutters.

SERVINGS
1

SERVING SIZE
2 toasted cheese people

Nutrition information for 1 serving

Calories	135
Total Fat	1 g
Saturated fat	0 g
Cholesterol	5 mg
Sodium	616 mg
Total carbohydrate	20 g
Fiber	4 g
Protein	11 g

Exchanges

1 Starch
1 Meat, very lean
1 Vegetable

Baked Potato Boats

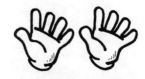

B is for baked potato.

INGREDIENTS

- **1** small baking potato (about 3 ounces)
- **1/4** teaspoon reduced-fat tub margarine
- **2** dashes salt
- **1** dash pepper
- **1** teaspoon fat-free milk
- **1** teaspoon bacon bits
- **1/2** (3/4-ounce) slice fat-free American cheese

EQUIPMENT

Measuring spoons

Cutting board

Knife

Plate

Potholders

Spoon (regular)

Small mixing bowl

Potato masher (or fork)

Toothpick

DO THIS FIRST

▌Check with an adult before you begin cooking and ask for help at the microwave/oven and with cutting.

▌Read through the whole recipe and make sure you have all of the ingredients and equipment you need.

DIRECTIONS

1 Bake potato in microwave at 100% power until tender (2–3 minutes) or in the oven at 425°F until tender (about 45 minutes).

2 Carefully cut cooked potato in half and allow it to cool enough to handle (about 10 minutes).

3 Using a spoon, scrape the inside of the potato into a bowl, leaving a 1/4-inch layer inside the skin.

4 Mash the potato pulp using a hand-held potato masher or fork. Add margarine, salt, and pepper, then mash again. Add fat-free milk and mash once more (add more or less milk to desired thickness).

5 Carefully spoon the mashed potato into the 2 potato skins.

6 Sprinkle both with bacon bits.

7 Heat briefly, if desired, in the microwave or oven.

8 Cut the cheese slice in half to make 2 squares. Hold each cheese square and carefully push a toothpick through the top side of the cheese slice, then back up through the under side of the cheese slice, making a sail. Repeat with the other cheese slice to make a second sail. Stick the cheese sails in the potato boats.

PREPARATION TIME
15 minutes (microwave)

COOLING TIME
10 minutes

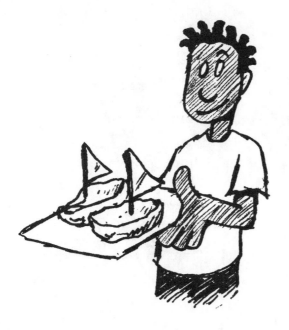

SERVINGS
1

SERVING SIZE
2 potato boats

Nutrition information for 1 serving

Calories	94
Total fat	1 g
Saturated fat	0 g
Cholesterol	3 mg
Sodium	223 mg
Total carbohydrate	16 g
Fiber	2 g
Protein	5 g

Exchanges

1 Starch

Cock-a-Doodle-Doo Spread

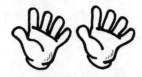

C is for chicken.

INGREDIENTS

- **2** ounces fat-free cream cheese (about 1/4 cup)
- **1** (16-ounce) container reduced-fat sour cream
- **1** (1-ounce) envelope ranch-style salad dressing mix
- **2** tablespoons finely grated carrot
- **1** (10-ounce) can 98% fat-free white chicken canned in water

DO THIS FIRST

- Check with an adult before you begin cooking and ask for help with using the grater, can opener, and electric mixer.
- Read through the whole recipe and make sure you have all of the ingredients and equipment you need.
- Grate enough carrot to make 2 tablespoons.

EQUIPMENT

Measuring spoons
Grater (optional)
Can opener
Electric mixer
Mixing bowl
Rubber spatula
Fork
Plastic wrap

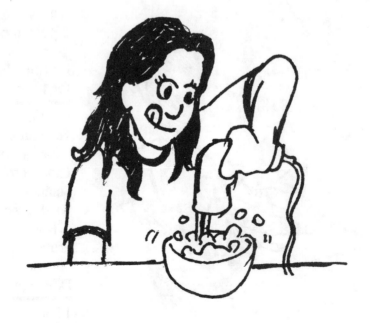

DIRECTIONS

1 Place cream cheese in a small mixing bowl. Using an electric mixer on the medium setting, whip cream cheese until fluffy. Scrape down bowl with a rubber spatula.

2 Whip in sour cream, then dressing mix, then carrot.

3 Open canned chicken, drain well, and break up chicken with a fork. Mix chicken into cream cheese mixture.

4 Cover and chill in the refrigerator for at least 2 hours to allow flavors to blend.

PREPARATION TIME
10 minutes

CHILLING TIME
2 hours

GOOD TO KNOW

▌ For convenience, purchase grated carrot from a grocery salad bar or prepackaged from the produce section.

▌ This is great as a spread on bread or low-fat snack crackers.

SERVINGS
13

SERVING SIZE
1/4 cup

Nutrition information for 1 serving

Calories 74
Total fat . . . . 3 g
    Saturated fat . . . . 2 g
Cholesterol . . . . 24 mg
Sodium . . . . 398 mg
Total carbohydrate . . . . . . 4 g
    Fiber . . . . 0 g
Protein . . . . 8 g

Exchanges

1 Meat, very lean
1 Fat

Crispy Chicken Drumsticks

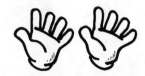

D is for drumstick.

INGREDIENTS

cooking spray

6 chicken drumsticks (about 2 pounds)

1/2 cup canned fried onions

1/2 cup cornflakes cereal

3 tablespoons spicy brown mustard

EQUIPMENT

Measuring spoons

Measuring cups

Baking sheet

Pan

Potholder

Strainer

Long-handled mixing spoon

Zip-top plastic bag

Rolling pin

Pie plate (shallow)

Pastry brush

DO THIS FIRST

▌ Check with an adult before you begin cooking and ask for help at the stove and oven.

▌ Read through the whole recipe and make sure you have all of the ingredients and equipment you need.

DIRECTIONS

1 Coat a baking sheet with cooking spray; set aside.

2 Place drumsticks in a pan and cover with water. Bring water to a boil over high heat, reduce heat to medium-high, and cook 20 minutes, or until chicken is no longer pink. Carefully drain off water.

3 Set cooked chicken aside and allow to cool (about 20 minutes). Remove skin and throw it away.

4 Preheat oven to 325°F.

5 Place fried onions and cornflakes cereal in a zip-top bag. Push air out of the bag, seal the bag, and crush fried onions and cereal in it by using a rolling pin. Pour crumbs into a shallow pan (like a pie plate); set aside.

6 Using a pastry brush, coat each chicken drumstick evenly with mustard, then put drumsticks one at a time into the crumbs and roll to coat with crumbs.

7 Place coated drumsticks on the baking sheet and pour remaining crumbs over them.

8 Bake for 12–15 minutes, or until heated through.

PREPARATION TIME
35 minutes

COOLING TIME
20 minutes

BAKING TIME
12–15 minutes

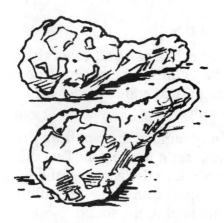

SERVINGS
6

SERVING SIZE
1 drumstick

**Nutrition information
for 1 serving**

Calories	124
Total fat	5 g
Saturated fat	1 g
Cholesterol	40 mg
Sodium	274 mg
Total carbohydrate	5 g
Fiber	0 g
Protein	14 g

Exchanges

1/2 Starch
2 Meat, lean

Stuffed Green Eggs with Ham

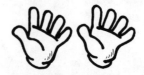

E is for egg.

INGREDIENTS

6 large eggs

1/4 cup reduced-fat mayonnaise

1 teaspoon coarse grain mustard

1/2 teaspoon fresh-squeezed lemon juice

4 drops green food coloring

1/8 teaspoon cayenne pepper sauce (such as Tabasco sauce)

1/8 teaspoon salt

1 teaspoon drained bottled horseradish (not horseradish sauce)

1/4 cup minced lean deli-slice ham (about 1 ounce or 4 paper-thin slices)

EQUIPMENT

Measuring cups

Measuring spoons

Knife

Cutting board

Pan

Potholder

Small mixing bowl

Fork

Long-handled mixing spoon

Spoon (regular)

Plastic wrap

DIRECTIONS

1 Place eggs in a pan and cover them with water. Bring the water to a boil over high heat and boil eggs for 20 minutes.

2 Carefully remove the pan from the heat and set it in the sink. Let cold water run into the pan over the eggs for a couple of minutes, or until the eggs are cool to the touch.

3 Peel cooled eggs and slice them in half. Remove yolks to a bowl and mash them with a fork so that there are no lumps.

4 Add mayonnaise, mustard, lemon juice, food coloring, cayenne pepper sauce, salt, and horseradish to the egg yolks; stir until well mixed.

5 Add ham and stir until ham is evenly mixed into the filling.

6 Spoon filling into egg whites.

7 Cover and refrigerate until serving time.

PREPARATION TIME
20 minutes

COOKING TIME
25 minutes

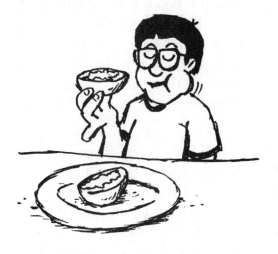

SERVES
12

SERVING
1 egg half

Nutrition information for 1 serving

Calories	58
Total fat	4 g
Saturated fat	1 g
Cholesterol	109 mg
Sodium	140 mg
Total carbohydrate	1 g
Fiber	0 g
Protein	4 g

Exchanges

1 Meat, lean

"Fun"due

F is for fondue.

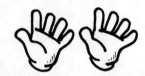

INGREDIENTS

1 cup Ragu cheese sauce

2 cups broccoli florets

2 cups snow pea pods

4 ounces cooked chicken breast cut into 1-inch chunks (try using frozen cooked chicken breast chunks or strips)

4 ounces cooked beef cut into 1-inch chunks (try using frozen cooked beef chunks or strips)

4 ounces French bread cut into 1-inch cubes, warmed if desired

1 cup grape or cherry tomatoes

EQUIPMENT

Knife

Cutting board

Measuring cups

Nonstick skillet (optional; to cook meat)

Microwave-safe dish with lid (or saucepan)

Large pan with lid

Potholder

Fondue pot (or crock-pot)

Serving tray

Bamboo skewers

DO THIS FIRST

- Check with an adult before you begin cooking and ask for help at the stove/ microwave and with cutting.
- Read through the whole recipe and make sure you have all of the ingredients and equipment you need.
- Cut up enough broccoli tops to make 2 cups.
- If not using precooked chicken, cook a 4-ounce chicken breast and cut into 1-inch chunks.
- If not using precooked beef, cook 4 ounces of lean steak or roast beef and cut into 1-inch chunks.
- Warm bread if desired and cut into 1-inch cubes.
- Slice tomatoes in half if young children will be eating the "fun"due.

DIRECTIONS

1 Place cheese sauce in a small microwave-safe dish, cover, and warm about 1 minute, or warm in a saucepan over low heat.

2 In a large pan, bring 2 cups water to a boil over high heat. When the water boils, add broccoli and snow pea pods.

3 Cover the pot with a lid and remove from the heat. Let the pot sit for 2 minutes, then carefully pour off all the water—watch out for steam. Set broccoli and snow pea pods aside.

4 If chicken and beef chunks are cold, warm in the microwave if desired.

5 To keep the cheese sauce warm during the "fun"due, pour it into a fondue pot or a small crock-pot on LOW heat.

6 Place broccoli, snow pea pods, chicken, beef, bread cubes, and tomatoes on a serving tray.

7 Use bamboo skewers as fondue sticks to spear pieces of food and dip them in the cheese sauce.

PREPARATION TIME
30 minutes

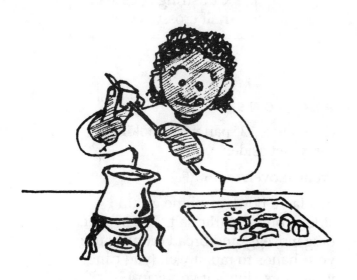

SERVINGS
4

SERVING SIZE
1/4 of recipe

**Nutrition information
for 1 serving**

Calories. 262
Total fat. . . . . 8 g
    Saturated fat . . . . 3 g
Cholesterol. . . . . 74 mg
Sodium . . . . 655 mg
Total carbohydrate. . . . . 23 g
    Fiber . . . . 3 g
Protein . . . . 25 g

Exchanges

1 Starch
3 Meat, lean
1 Vegetable

Mini Meat Loaf Treasures

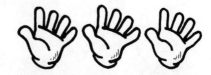

G is for ground beef.

INGREDIENTS

cooking spray

1 pound ground sirloin

1 tablespoon dried minced onion

1/2 teaspoon garlic salt

1/4 teaspoon salt

1/8 teaspoon black pepper

1/2 teaspoon dried leaf oregano

1 large egg, beaten

1/4 cup plain dry bread crumbs

2 (1-ounce) sticks string cheese, cut in half crosswise

1/2 cup pizza sauce

EQUIPMENT

Whisk (or fork)

Small mixing bowl

Knife

Cutting board

Measuring cups

Measuring spoons

9" x 13" pan

Large mixing bowl

Latex gloves (optional)

Potholder

Spoon (optional)

DO THIS FIRST

▎ Check with an adult before you begin cooking and ask for help with the oven.

▎ Read through the whole recipe and make sure you have all of the ingredients and equipment you need.

▎ Break the egg into a small bowl and beat with a fork or whisk.

▎ Crumble up stale bread to make 1/4 cup crumbs if not using prepackaged bread crumbs.

▎ Cut string cheese in half crosswise.

DIRECTIONS

1 Coat a 9" x 13" pan with cooking spray; set aside.

2 Preheat oven to 350°F.

3 In a large bowl, combine ground sirloin, onion, garlic salt, salt, pepper, oregano, egg, and bread crumbs; use your hands to mix it well (you can wear latex gloves if you want).

4 Split the meat mixture into 4 equal parts. Shape each into a rectangle around one piece of string cheese— the cheese should be completely covered with meat.

5 Place meat loaves 1 1/2 to 2 inches apart in the pan. Bake for 30 minutes, or until the meat is no longer pink inside (cheese may melt out of the meat loaves slightly).

6 Carefully drain or spoon off any grease, then pour pizza sauce evenly over meat loaves to cover the sides.

7 Bake 15 minutes more.

PREPARATION TIME
20 minutes

BAKING TIME
45 minutes

G O O D   T O   K N O W

For smaller appetites, cut cooked meat loaves in half.

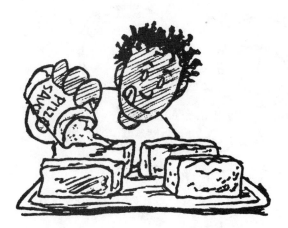

SERVINGS
4 meat loaves

SERVING SIZE
1 meat loaf

Nutrition information for 1 serving

Calories	256
Total fat	10 g
Saturated fat	4 g
Cholesterol	130 mg
Sodium	796 mg
Total carbohydrate	9 g
Fiber	0 g
Protein	30 g

Exchanges

1/2 Starch
4 Meat, lean

Ham Mouse Face

H is for ham.

INGREDIENTS

1 (3-ounce) slice of fully-cooked ham
(about 1/4 inch thick)

2 radish slices

2 black or green olive slices
ketchup

6 (2-inch) pieces of chives

EQUIPMENT

Knife

Cutting board

Small cookie
(or biscuit) cutter

Large cookie
(or biscuit) cutter

Plate

DO THIS FIRST

▌ Check with an adult
before you begin
cooking and ask for
help with cutting.

▌ Read through the
whole recipe and
make sure you have
all of the ingredients
and equipment you
need.

▌ Cut 2 radish slices,
2 olive slices, and
6 pieces of chives
2 inches long each.

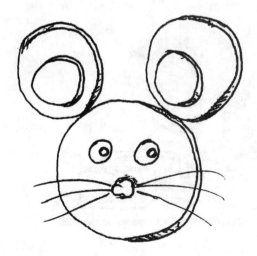

DIRECTIONS

1 Lay the ham on the cutting board. Cut 1 large and 2 small circles out of the ham using the cookie or biscuit cutters. Save leftover pieces of ham for another use.

2 Place the large ham circle in the center of your plate. This is the mouse's head.

3 Place the 2 small ham circles at the top of the large ham circle for the mouse's ears.

4 Lay the 2 radish slices in the center of the 2 small ham circles to make the inside of the mouse's ears.

5 Use the olive slices to make eyes.

6 Make a nose with ketchup and lay three chives on each side of the ketchup for whiskers.

PREPARATION TIME
5 minutes

SERVINGS
1

SERVING SIZE
1 mouse face

Nutrition information for 1 serving

Calories	90
Total fat	3 g
Saturated fat	1 g
Cholesterol	31 mg
Sodium	759 mg
Total carbohydrate	1 g
Fiber	0 g
Protein	14 g

Exchanges

2 Meat, lean

Lasagna Rollers

I is for Italian entrée.

INGREDIENTS

cooking spray

1 pound ground sirloin

1 (26-ounce) jar light spaghetti sauce

8 ounces uncooked lasagna noodles (9 noodles)

1 large egg

1 (16-ounce) container fat-free cottage cheese

8 tablespoons grated Parmesan cheese

1/8 teaspoon black pepper

1 cup (4 ounces) finely shredded part-skim mozzarella cheese

EQUIPMENT

Measuring spoons

Measuring cups

9" x 13" pan

Nonstick skillet

Metal spatula

Potholder

Strainer

Pan

Large mixing bowl

Fork

Long-handled mixing spoon

DO THIS FIRST

▌ Check with an adult before you begin cooking and ask for help at the stove and oven.

▌ Read through the whole recipe and make sure you have all of the ingredients and equipment you need.

DIRECTIONS

1 Preheat oven to 350°F.

2 Coat a 9" x 13" baking pan with cooking spray; set aside.

3 Place ground sirloin in a large non-stick skillet and cook over medium-high heat until no longer pink (about 6–7 minutes). Carefully drain off any grease.

4 Add spaghetti sauce to meat, reduce heat to low, cover, and cook for 15 minutes.

5 Meanwhile, cook lasagna noodles according to package directions, omitting any salt.

6 Carefully drain noodles. Rinse with cold water and drain again; set aside.

7 Crack egg into a large bowl and beat with a fork until frothy. Stir in cottage cheese, Parmesan cheese, and black pepper.

8 Lay lasagna noodles flat on a clean counter. Spread the length of each lasagna noodle with a little less than 1/4 cup of the cottage cheese mixture, then spread about 1/4 cup of the meat mixture down the center of the noodle over the cottage cheese mixture.

9 Loosely roll each lasagna noodle up from one end to the other and using a metal spatula place seam-side down in the pan coated with cooking spray. Place lasagna rollers side by side in the pan. Any filling that leaks out when rolling up the lasagna noodles can be spooned into the baking pan around the lasagna rollers.

10 Spoon remaining meat sauce over the rollers. Sprinkle each roller with mozzarella cheese.

11 Bake uncovered for 25–30 minutes, or until cheese is melted and the sauce is bubbly.

PREPARATION TIME
30 minutes

BAKING TIME
25–30 minutes

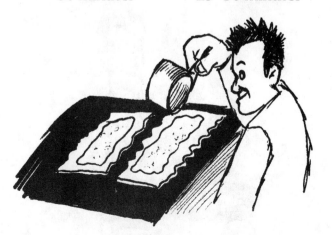

GOOD TO KNOW

Leftovers re-heat well!

SERVINGS
9

SERVING SIZE
1 roller

Nutrition information for 1 serving

Calories 289	
Total fat . . . . 8 g	
Saturated fat . . . . 4 g	
Cholesterol . . . . 66 mg	
Sodium . . . . 725 mg	
Total carbohydrate . . . . . 29 g	
Fiber . . . . 3 g	
Protein . . . . 25 g	

Exchanges

1 1/2 Starch
2 Meat, lean
1 Vegetable
1/2 Fat

Hoedown Johnnycakes

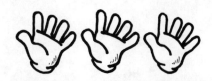

J is for johnnycake.

INGREDIENTS

1 (6.5-ounce) package corn bread mix that requires only the addition of water (as stated on the corn bread mix package)

cooking spray

1 (15-ounce) can pinto beans

1/2 cup water

1/4 cup + **2** tablespoons finely shredded reduced-fat cheddar cheese

2 1/4 cups chopped lettuce

1/2 cup + **1** tablespoon finely chopped tomato

EQUIPMENT

Can opener

Grater

Knife

Cutting board

Measuring cups

Measuring spoons

Large mixing bowl

Small pan

Fork

Nonstick skillet (or griddle)

Metal spatula

Plate

Spoon

DO THIS FIRST

▌ Check with an adult before you begin cooking and ask for help with the can opener, grater, cutting, and at the stove.

▌ Read through the whole recipe and make sure you have all of the ingredients and equipment you need.

▌ If not using prepackaged shredded cheese, grate enough reduced-fat cheddar cheese to make 1/4 cup + 2 tablespoons.

▌ If not using prepackaged chopped lettuce, finely chop enough lettuce to make 2 1/4 cups.

▌ Finely chop enough tomato to make 1/2 cup + 1 tablespoon.

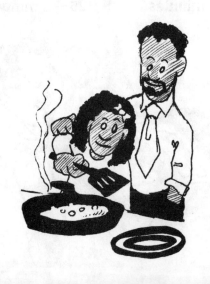

DIRECTIONS

1 Prepare corn bread mix batter according to package directions; set aside.

2 Place pinto beans in a small pan. Mash about 1/3 of them with a fork. Add 1/2 cup water (use more for a thinner sauce or less for a thicker sauce) and warm over medium heat, stirring frequently, until a sauce forms. Turn heat down to low.

3 Coat a nonstick skillet or griddle with cooking spray and warm over medium heat.

4 Make johnnycakes as you would pancakes, by pouring 1/8 cup of batter onto the skillet for each johnnycake. Cook about 2–3 minutes, or until the tops of the johnnycakes bubble. Turn johnnycakes over with a spatula and continue cooking 1–2 minutes more, or until done. (Reduce the heat if they brown too fast). Recoat the skillet or griddle with cooking spray between batches.

5 Remove cooked johnnycakes to a plate and cover to keep them warm until the cooking is finished.

6 To serve, place 1 johnnycake on each plate. Spoon about 1/4 cup beans over it then sprinkle with 2 teaspoons cheese, 1/4 cup lettuce, and 1 tablespoon tomato. Serve right away.

PREPARATION TIME
40 minutes

GOOD TO KNOW

You can use other corn bread mixes. We chose one that just uses water to keep the recipe simple.

SERVINGS
9

SERVING SIZE
1 johnnycake

**Nutrition information
for 1 serving**

Calories. 136
Total fat. . . . . 3 g
 Saturated fat . . . . 1 g
Cholesterol. . . . . 4 mg
Sodium . . . . 438 mg
Total carbohydrate. . . . . 23 g
 Fiber . . . . 3 g
Protein. . . . . 5 g

Exchanges

1 1/2 Starch
1/2 Fat

Bean Spread Cracker Stackers

K is for kidney bean.

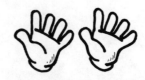

INGREDIENTS

1 (15-ounce) can kidney beans, rinsed and drained

2 teaspoons (or 2 cloves) crushed garlic

1/2 teaspoon ground cumin

1/2 teaspoon cayenne pepper sauce (such as Tabasco sauce)

1 tablespoon apple cider vinegar

1 tablespoon sour cream

2 teaspoons dried parsley

1/2 teaspoon salt

90 baked whole-wheat snack crackers (such as Triscuits)

EQUIPMENT

Can opener

Blender (or food processor)

Strainer

Garlic press (optional)

Measuring spoons

Rubber spatula

Airtight container

Spoon

DO THIS FIRST

▮ Check with an adult before you begin cooking and ask for help with the can opener and blender/food processor.

▮ Read through the whole recipe and make sure you have all of the ingredients and equipment you need.

▮ Open the can of kidney beans, rinse, and drain well.

▮ If not using bottled crushed garlic, then use a garlic press or dull knife to crush 2 cloves of garlic.

DIRECTIONS

1 Place all of the ingredients except the crackers in a blender or food processor and process until smooth. If needed, turn off blender or food processor, remove the lid, and scrape down the sides with a rubber spatula. Remember to put the lid back on before turning machine back on.

2 Cover bean spread and refrigerate at least one hour to allow flavors to blend.

3 Make stackers by spreading 1 cracker with 1 teaspoon bean dip, topping it with a second cracker, spreading the second cracker with 1 teaspoon bean dip, and then topping it with a third cracker.

4 Repeat to make 30 stackers.

5 Serve stackers right away.

PREPARATION TIME
25 minutes

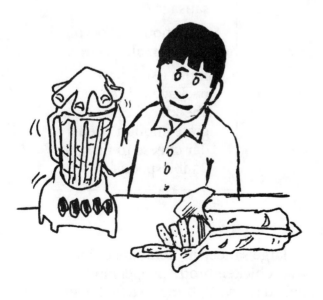

SERVINGS
30

SERVING SIZE
1 stacker

**Nutrition information
for 1 serving**

Calories	67
Total fat	2 g
Saturated fat	1 g
Cholesterol	0 mg
Sodium	135 mg
Total carbohydrate	11 g
Fiber	2 g
Protein	2 g

Exchanges

1 Starch

Leapin' Linguini

L is for linguini.

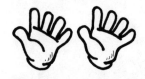

INGREDIENTS

1 teaspoon dried minced onion

1 teaspoon (or 1 clove) minced garlic

1 (14 1/2-ounce) can fat-free reduced-sodium chicken broth

1/8 teaspoon black pepper

4 ounces low-fat smoked sausage (such as Healthy Choice smoked sausage), thinly sliced

5 ounces uncooked linguini (about a handful of uncooked linguini broken into 1-inch pieces)

2 cups fresh broccoli florets

1/4 cup + **2** tablespoons light sour cream

2 tablespoons finely shredded cheddar cheese

EQUIPMENT

Knife

Cutting board

Grater (optional)

Can opener

Measuring spoons

Measuring cups

Large saucepan with lid

Long-handled mixing spoon

DO THIS FIRST

▌Check with an adult before you begin cooking and ask for help with the cutting, can opener, grater, and at the stove.

▌Read through the whole recipe and make sure you have all of the ingredients and equipment you need.

▌Very finely chop 1 peeled garlic clove, if not using bottled minced garlic.

▌Thinly slice smoked sausage.

▌Cut enough broccoli tops to make 2 cups.

▌If not using pre-packaged shredded cheddar cheese, grate enough cheddar cheese to make 2 tablespoons.

DIRECTIONS

1 In a large saucepan, combine onion, garlic, chicken broth, pepper, and smoked sausage; bring to a boil over high heat.

2 Add linguini; stir to mix. Return to a boil, then reduce heat to medium-low and simmer, covered, for 7–8 minutes; carefully remove the lid and stir periodically.

3 Add broccoli, cover, and simmer 5–6 minutes more, or until pasta is tender.

4 Remove pan from heat. Stir in sour cream and toss pasta to coat well.

5 Spoon pasta onto plates or into serving dish. Sprinkle with cheese.

PREPARATION TIME
30 minutes

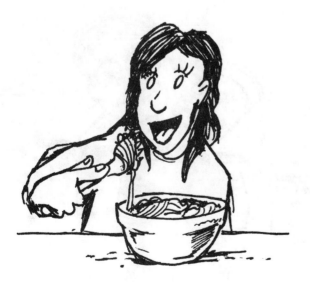

SERVINGS
3

SERVING SIZE
1 heaping cup

**Nutrition information
for 1 serving**

Calories 307
Total fat . . . . 7 g
    Saturated fat . . . . 3 g
Cholesterol . . . . 31 mg
Sodium . . . . 717 mg
Total carbohydrate . . . . . 45 g
    Fiber . . . . 3 g
Protein . . . . 17 g

Exchanges

2 1/2 Starch
1 Meat, lean
1 Vegetable
1/2 Fat

Wacky Tomato Macky

M is for macaroni.

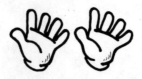

INGREDIENTS

- **1** (7-ounce) box elbow macaroni
- **2** (14 1/2-ounce) cans diced tomatoes seasoned with basil, garlic, and oregano; undrained
- **1/8** teaspoon pepper
- **1** teaspoon corn oil
- **1** tablespoon grated Parmesan cheese

EQUIPMENT

Can opener

Measuring spoons

Pan

Strainer

Long-handled
  mixing spoon

DO THIS FIRST

- Check with an adult before you begin cooking and ask for help at the stove and with the can opener.
- Read through the whole recipe and make sure you have all of the ingredients and equipment you need.

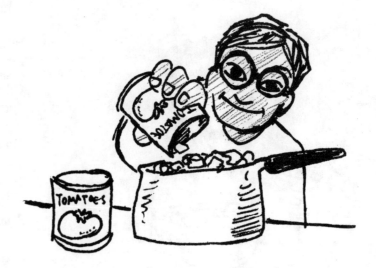

DIRECTIONS

1 Cook macaroni according to package directions, omitting any salt. Drain well.

2 Add tomatoes, pepper, and oil to macaroni.

3 Cook uncovered over medium-low heat for 15 minutes, or until tomatoes are cooked down.

4 Spoon into a serving dish and sprinkle evenly with Parmesan cheese.

PREPARATION TIME
30 minutes

GOOD TO KNOW

You can make this recipe using other shaped pasta, such as wagon wheel or bow tie.

SERVINGS
13

SERVING SIZE
1/2 cup

**Nutrition information
for 1 serving**

Calories 84
Total fat . . . . 1 g
   Saturated fat . . . . 0 g
Cholesterol . . . . 1 mg
Sodium . . . . 336 mg
Total carbohydrate . . . . . 16 g
   Fiber . . . . 1 g
Protein . . . . 3 g

Exchanges

1 Starch

Ranch-Style Nachos

N is for nachos.

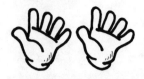

INGREDIENTS

16 baked tortilla chips (about 1 ounce)

3 ounces frozen cooked chicken breast strips or chunks, thawed

1/4 cup (1 ounce) finely shredded reduced-fat cheddar cheese

1/2 cup chopped tomato

2 tablespoons light ranch-style dressing

EQUIPMENT

Grater (optional)

Knife

Cutting board

Measuring spoons

Measuring cups

Baking sheet

Fork

Potholder

Plate

DO THIS FIRST

▌ Check with an adult before you begin cooking and ask for help at the oven and with the grater.

▌ Read through the whole recipe and make sure you have all of the ingredients and equipment you need.

▌ Thaw the cooked chicken breast strips or chunks.

▌ If not using pre-packaged shredded cheese, grate enough reduced-fat cheddar cheese to make 1/4 cup.

▌ Chop enough tomato to make 1/2 cup.

DIRECTIONS

1 Preheat oven to 350°F.

2 Place tortilla chips closely together in a single layer on a baking sheet; set aside.

3 Using a fork, shred thawed chicken breast strips or chunks. Sprinkle shredded meat evenly over tortilla chips.

4 Sprinkle cheese evenly over chicken.

5 Bake for 5–7 minutes, or until cheese melts. Watch closely and remove nachos from the oven if chips begin to brown.

6 Transfer nachos to a serving dish and sprinkle them with chopped tomato, then drizzle with dressing.

PREPARATION TIME
15 minutes

BAKING TIME
5–7 minutes

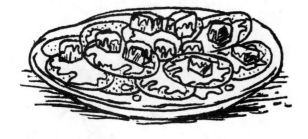

SERVINGS
2

SERVING SIZE
8 nachos

Nutrition information for 1 serving

Calories	215
Total fat	9 g
Saturated fat	3 g
Cholesterol	46 mg
Sodium	395 mg
Total carbohydrate	16 g
Fiber	2 g
Protein	19 g

Exchanges

1 Starch
2 Meat, lean
1/2 Fat

Hidden Treasure Omelet

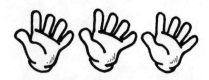

O is for omelet.

INGREDIENTS

cooking spray

3 teaspoons reduced-fat margarine, divided

1/4 cup frozen shredded hash brown potatoes, thawed

2 patties (about 1 ounce) cooked low-fat breakfast sausage (such as Healthy Choice)

1 large egg + **2** large egg whites

2 teaspoons fat-free milk

2 dashes pepper

2 dashes salt

2 tablespoons finely shredded reduced-fat cheddar cheese

DO THIS FIRST

▌ Check with an adult before you begin cooking and ask for help at the stove, and with cutting and the grater.

▌ Read through the whole recipe and make sure you have all of the ingredients and equipment you need.

▌ Thaw hash browns.

▌ If not using pre-packaged shredded cheese, grate enough reduced-fat cheddar cheese to make 2 tablespoons.

EQUIPMENT

Grater (optional)

Knife

Cutting board

Measuring spoons

Measuring cups

Small nonstick skillet with lid

Metal spatula

Plate

Medium mixing bowl

Whisk

Spoon

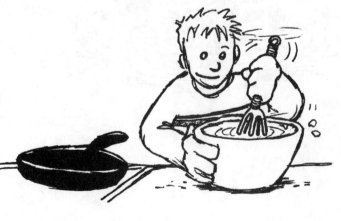

DIRECTIONS

1 Coat a small nonstick skillet with cooking spray, then melt 1 teaspoon margarine in the skillet over medium heat. Add hash brown potatoes. Cook and stir until potatoes are tender and light golden, about 4–5 minutes. Remove hash browns from skillet and cover to keep them warm.

2 Chop sausage into little pieces and warm in the microwave 20–30 seconds; set aside and cover to keep warm.

3 In a bowl, whisk together egg, egg whites, milk, pepper, and salt; set aside.

4 In the same skillet used in step 1, melt the remaining 2 teaspoons margarine over medium-low heat. Rotate the pan to coat the bottom with margarine.

5 Pour egg mixture into the skillet. As the egg begins to cook and set, carefully lift the edges of the omelet with a spatula so that the uncooked egg flows underneath (tilt the skillet if needed).

6 When the omelet is fully cooked, spoon cooked hash browns over half of omelet. Top them with the sausage, then cheese.

7 Loosen omelet with a spatula and fold it in half. Use spatula to remove omelet from the skillet.

PREPARATION TIME
20 minutes

GOOD TO KNOW

An omelet pan is handy, although not necessary, for this recipe.

SERVINGS
2

SERVING SIZE
1/2 omelet

Nutrition information for 1 serving

Calories	145
Total fat	8 g
Saturated fat	3 g
Cholesterol	120 mg
Sodium	352 mg
Total carbohydrate	7 g
Fiber	0 g
Protein	12 g

Exchanges

1/2 Starch
2 Meat, lean

Monkey's uncle Pancakes

P is for pancakes.

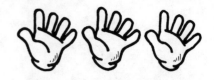

INGREDIENTS

3/4 cup rolled oats

2 teaspoons whole-wheat flour

1 1/2 teaspoons baking powder

1/8 teaspoon cinnamon

3/4 cup fat-free milk

1 egg white

1 1/2 teaspoons corn oil

1/2 medium (6-ounce) banana, mashed

cooking spray

EQUIPMENT

Fork

Measuring cups

Measuring spoons

Blender (or Food processor)

Long-handled mixing spoon

Large nonstick skillet (or Griddle)

Metal spatula

Plate

DO THIS FIRST

▮ Check with an adult before you begin cooking and ask for help with the blender and at the stove.

▮ Read through the whole recipe and make sure you have all of the ingredients and equipment you need.

▮ Mash banana with a fork.

DIRECTIONS

1 Place oats, whole-wheat flour, baking powder, and cinnamon in a blender or food processor. Cover tightly and blend or process until powdery, like flour.

2 Add milk, egg white, corn oil, and banana. Use the long-handled spoon to stir down to the bottom of the blender to loosen the flour. Remove the spoon, cover tightly, and blend until mixed—the batter will be thin.

3 Let batter sit for 5 minutes—it will thicken some.

4 Coat the large nonstick skillet or griddle with cooking spray. Warm skillet over medium heat.

5 Pour a 1/4 cup batter per pancake into skillet and cook until the tops of the pancakes begin to bubble (about 3–4 minutes). Using a metal spatula, turn pancakes over and cook the other side until done (about 2–3 minutes). Recoat skillet with cooking spray between batches.

PREPARATION TIME
30 minutes

GOOD TO KNOW

Leftover pancakes are tasty when re-heated in the microwave!

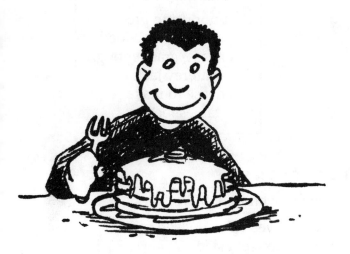

SERVINGS
5

SERVING SIZE
1 pancake

**Nutrition information
for 1 serving**

Calories	90
Total fat	2 g
Saturated fat	0 g
Cholesterol	1 mg
Sodium	140 mg
Total carbohydrate	14 g
Fiber	2 g
Protein	4 g

Exchanges

1 Starch

Mini Quiches

Q is for quiche.

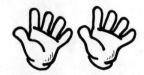

INGREDIENTS

1 (2.1-ounce) package frozen fully-cooked mini fillo dough shells, thawed (15 shells)

1/4 cup liquid egg substitute

2 tablespoons fat-free milk

2 dashes salt

1 dash black pepper

3 tablespoons finely chopped Canadian bacon (about 1 ounce)

2 tablespoons frozen corn, thawed

1 tablespoon finely chopped green onion

3 tablespoons finely shredded Monterey Jack cheese

EQUIPMENT

Knife

Cutting board

Grater (optional)

Measuring cups

Measuring spoons

Mini-muffin tins

2 small mixing bowls

Whisk

Spoon

Foil (optional)

Potholder

DO THIS FIRST

▌ Check with an adult before you begin cooking and ask for help at the oven and with cutting.

▌ Read through the whole recipe and make sure you have all of the ingredients and equipment you need.

▌ Thaw the fillo shells and corn.

▌ Finely chop Canadian bacon.

▌ Finely chop enough green onions to make 1 tablespoon.

▌ If not using pre-packaged shredded cheese, grate enough Monterey Jack cheese to make 3 tablespoons.

DIRECTIONS

1 Preheat oven to 350°F.

2 Place thawed fillo shells in mini muffin tins; set aside.

3 In a small bowl, whisk together egg substitute, milk, salt, and pepper; set aside.

4 In a separate bowl, stir together Canadian bacon, corn, green onion, and cheese. Spoon meat mixture into each shell, filling to the top—do not pack it down.

5 Pour the egg mixture over the meat mixture in each shell, filling nearly to the top edge of each shell.

6 Bake 13–15 minutes, or until puffed and a knife inserted in the center comes out clean. Lay foil over top of quiches if the shells begin to get too brown.

PREPARATION TIME
15 minutes

BAKING TIME
13–15 minutes

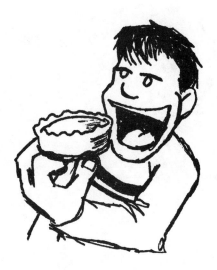

GOOD TO KNOW

You can substitute lean ham in place of the Canadian bacon.

SERVES
5

SERVING SIZE
3 quiches

**Nutrition information
for 1 serving**

Calories	105
Total fat	5 g
Saturated fat	1 g
Cholesterol	7 mg
Sodium	167 mg
Total carbohydrate	9 g
Fiber	0 g
Protein	5 g

Exchanges

1/2 Starch
1 Meat, medium fat

Red Rice

R is for rice.

INGREDIENTS

3/4 cup 100% vegetable juice

1/4 cup fat-free, reduced-sodium chicken broth

1 cup uncooked instant white rice

EQUIPMENT

Measuring cups

Large saucepan with lid

Long-handled mixing spoon

Fork

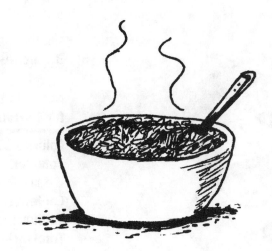

DIRECTIONS

1 Place vegetable juice and chicken broth in a pan, cover with lid, and bring to a boil over high heat.

2 Stir in rice, cover pan again with lid, and return to a boil for 30 seconds. Remove pan from the heat and let it stand, covered, for 5 minutes.

3 Remove lid from pan carefully (watch for steam) and fluff rice with a fork.

PREPARATION TIME
10 minutes

GOOD TO KNOW

Be sure to use instant white rice.

SERVINGS
4

SERVING SIZE
1/2 cup

Nutrition information for 1 serving

Calories	101
Total fat	0 g
Saturated fat	0 g
Cholesterol	0 mg
Sodium	150 mg
Total carbohydrate	22 g
Fiber	1 g
Protein	2 g

Exchanges

1 1/2 Starch

Saucy Spaghetti Squash

S is for spaghetti squash.

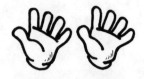

INGREDIENTS

1 spaghetti squash (about 1 1/4 pounds)
1 (14-ounce) jar spaghetti sauce
1/4 cup grated Parmesan cheese

EQUIPMENT

Knife

Cutting board

Measuring cups

Microwave-safe dish

Potholders

Spoon

Baking Pan

Fork

Microwave-safe plastic wrap (optional)

Pan with lid

Serving dish

DIRECTIONS

1 Preheat oven to 350°F.

2 Place whole squash in a microwave-safe dish and cook in the microwave for 5 minutes to soften the skin. Remove squash from the microwave with potholders.

3 Carefully cut squash in half lengthwise and scoop out any seeds.

4 Turn squash cut side down on a baking pan and bake 50–60 minutes, or until the squash is tender when pierced with a fork. (Alternately, place the squash cut side down in 1/4 cup water in a microwave-safe dish, cover with microwave-safe plastic wrap, and cook 8–10 minutes, or until tender when pierced with a fork.)

5 Meanwhile, place spaghetti sauce in a pan, cover with a lid, and warm over medium heat.

6 Run the prongs of fork along the length of the cut-side of the cooked squash to loosen spaghetti-like strands. Continue until you reach the hard peel of the squash.

7 Scoop squash strands into a serving dish.

8 Top with spaghetti sauce and sprinkle evenly with Parmesan cheese.

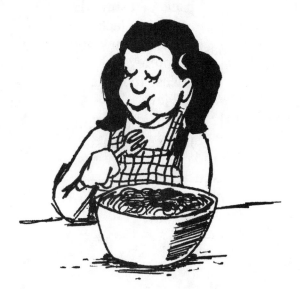

PREPARATION TIME
20 minutes

BAKING TIME
50–60 minutes (oven)
8–10 minutes (microwave)

GOOD TO KNOW

The squash peel is very tough, so be sure to ask an adult for help cutting the raw squash in half.

SERVES
12

SERVING SIZE
1/2 cup

Nutrition information for 1 serving

Calories	54
Total fat	2 g
Saturated fat	1 g
Cholesterol	3 mg
Sodium	211 mg
Total carbohydrate	7 g
Fiber	2 g
Protein	2 g

Exchanges

1/2 Starch
1/2 Fat

Buffalo Soft Tacos

T is for taco.

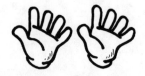

INGREDIENTS

1/3 cup mild cayenne pepper sauce (such as Frank's Red Hot Sauce, not Tabasco sauce)

1 teaspoon corn oil

2 cups (about 10 ounces) diced cooked chicken breast

4 (8-inch) flour tortillas, warmed if desired

1/2 cup (2 ounces) finely shredded Monterey Jack cheese

1 cup finely chopped lettuce

2 tablespoons + **2** teaspoons light ranch-style dressing

EQUIPMENT

Skillet (optional; to cook chicken)

Grater (optional)

Knife

Cutting board

Measuring cups

Measuring spoons

Zip-top bag

Microwave-safe dish with lid (or pan)

Spoon

DO THIS FIRST

▌ Check with an adult before you begin cooking and ask for help with cutting and at the stove/ microwave.

▌ Read through the whole recipe and make sure you have all of the ingredients and equipment you need.

▌ If not using frozen, fully-cooked chicken, cook chicken breast and chop it to make 2 cups.

▌ If not using pre-packaged shredded Monterey Jack cheese, grate enough Monterey Jack cheese to make 1/2 cup.

▌ Finely chop enough lettuce to make 1 cup.

DIRECTIONS

1 Put cayenne pepper sauce and oil in a large zip-top bag. Add cooked chicken, seal bag, and shake to coat chicken well. Refrigerate for 30 minutes to allow chicken to marinate.

2 Pour chicken and sauce in a microwave-safe dish, cover, and heat 2 minutes or until hot (or pour chicken and marinade in a pan and warm on the stove over medium heat).

3 Lay 4 flour tortillas on the counter. Spoon 1/4 of chicken in the center of each one. Drizzle with the warm marinade if you want to. Top each with 1/4 of the cheese and 1/4 of lettuce. Drizzle each with 1/4 dressing.

4 Fold each taco in half, or roll it up. Slice in half if you want to.

PREPARATION TIME
20 minutes

MARINATING TIME
30 minutes

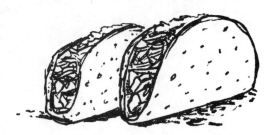

SERVES
4

SERVING SIZE
1 taco

Nutrition information for 1 serving

Calories	351
Total fat	13 g
Saturated fat	5 g
Cholesterol	72 mg
Sodium	1220 mg
Total carbohydrate	26 g
Fiber	2 g
Protein	30 g

Exchanges

1 1/2 Starch
4 Meat, lean

Under the Sea Submarine

U is for under the sea.

INGREDIENTS

1/4 cup tuna salad

1 hot dog bun

2 tomato slices

1 sandwich-sliced dill pickle

1 (3/4-ounce) slice fat-free American cheese

EQUIPMENT

Knife

Cutting board

Butter knife

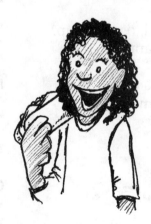

DIRECTIONS

1 Spread tuna salad on the bottom half of the hot dog bun.

2 Top with tomato slices and pickle slice.

3 Cut cheese slice in half diagonally to make 2 triangles; lay cheese triangles over the pickle slice.

4 Top with other half of bun.

PREPARATION TIME
5 minutes

GOOD TO KNOW

You can buy tuna salad or make your own tuna salad using low-fat mayonnaise.

SERVES
4

SERVING SIZE
1 taco

Nutrition information for 1 serving

Calories	260
Total fat	7 g
Saturated fat	1 g
Cholesterol	10 mg
Sodium	880 mg
Total carbohydrate	31 g
Fiber	2 g
Protein	17 g

Exchanges

2 Starch
2 Meat, very lean
1 Fat

Scout's Honor One-Pot-Pasta

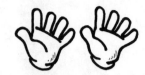

V is for vermicelli.

INGREDIENTS

3 1/2 cups water

4 ounces uncooked vermicelli pasta (a handful about 1 1/4" wide)

1 tablespoon dried minced onion

1 dash crushed red pepper flakes

1/4 teaspoon dried leaf oregano

1/4 teaspoon garlic powder

1 (24-ounce) package instant tomato with basil soup mix (such as Knorr)

1 (5-ounce) can chunk chicken breast in water, drained and flaked

2 teaspoons grated Parmesan cheese

EQUIPMENT

Can opener

Small mixing bowl

Fork

Grater (optional)

Measuring cups

Measuring spoons

Deep pan

Long-handled mixing spoon

Serving bowls

DO THIS FIRST

▌ Check with an adult before you begin cooking and ask for help at the stove and with the can opener and grater.

▌ Read through the whole recipe and make sure you have all of the ingredients and equipment you need.

▌ Open the can of chicken and drain well. Put chicken in a small bowl and flake it with a fork.

▌ If not using pre-packaged grated Parmesan cheese, grate 2 teaspoons of fresh Parmesan.

DIRECTIONS

1 Place water in a deep pan and bring to a boil over high heat. Add vermicelli pasta, onion, red pepper flakes, oregano, and garlic powder. Stir to separate pasta.

2 Reduce heat to medium-high and cook uncovered for 5–7 minutes, or until pasta is tender (do not drain pasta).

3 Reduce heat to medium-low, add soup mix, and stir well, breaking up clumps of soup mix with the spoon.

4 Cook 4 minutes longer; stir occasionally.

5 Stir in chicken and heat 1 minute more.

6 Spoon 1/2 cup into each bowl and sprinkle lightly with Parmesan cheese.

PREPARATION TIME
25 minutes

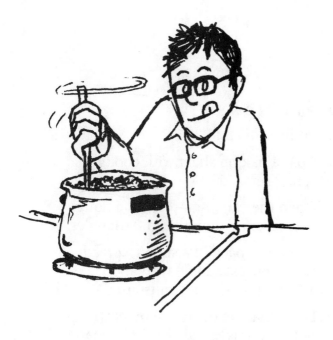

SERVES
7

SERVING SIZE
1/2 cup

Nutrition information for 1 serving

Calories	122
Total fat	2 g
Saturated fat	1 g
Cholesterol	11 mg
Sodium	490 mg
Total carbohydrate	18 g
Fiber	1 g
Protein	8 g

Exchanges

1 Starch
1 Meat, very lean

wild wrapped wieners

W is for wiener.

INGREDIENTS

cooking spray

1 (8-ounce) can reduced-fat crescent roll dough

1 tablespoon + **1** teaspoon honey mustard

4 (3/4-ounce) slices fat-free American cheese

8 low-fat beef wieners (such as Healthy Choice)

EQUIPMENT

Knife

Cutting board

Measuring spoons

Baking sheet

Spoon

Potholders

DO THIS FIRST

▌ Check with an adult before you begin cooking and ask for help at the oven.

▌ Read through the whole recipe and make sure you have all of the ingredients and equipment you need.

▌ Cut each slice of American cheese diagonally to make 2 triangles.

DIRECTIONS

1 Preheat oven to 375°F.

2 Coat a baking sheet with cooking spray; set aside.

3 Open the can of crescent roll dough and separate dough into 8 triangles.

4 Using the back of a spoon, spread each dough triangle with about 1/2 teaspoon honey mustard.

5 Lay a triangle of cheese on each dough triangle, matching the shapes together.

6 Lay a wiener across the bottom of each dough triangle and roll it up in the dough.

7 Place wrapped wieners 2 inches apart on the baking sheet and bake for 12–15 minutes, or until dough is golden and cooked.

PREPARATION TIME
15 minutes

BAKING TIME
12–15 minutes

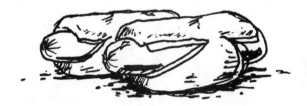

SERVINGS
8
SERVING SIZE
1 wiener

**Nutrition information
for 1 serving**

Calories	188
Total fat	7 g
Saturated fat	2 g
Cholesterol	22 mg
Sodium	822 mg
Total carbohydrate	20 g
Fiber	1 g
Protein	11 g

Exchanges

1 Starch
1 Meat, lean
1 Fat

Pasta Pictures

X is for X-tra special projects.

WHAT YOU'LL NEED

- Medium-sized bowls of water
- Red, yellow, and blue food coloring
- A variety of shapes of uncooked pasta—wheels, shells, bow ties, circles, tubes, and elbows
- Spoons
- Paper towels
- White glue
- Cardboard

WHAT YOU'LL DO

1 Mix a few drops of food coloring in each bowl of water. Mixing red, yellow and blue in various combinations will give you a wide variety of colors.

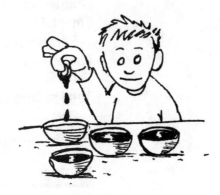

2 Drop uncooked pasta into the water for a minute or two, then remove with a spoon and dry on a paper towel.

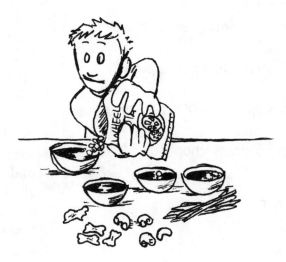

3 Use white glue to paste pasta to cardboard, making pictures such as animals, flowers, or interesting designs.

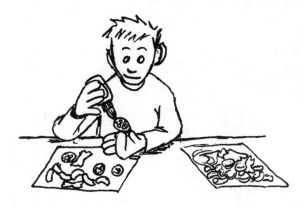

Yummy Yams

Y is for yams.

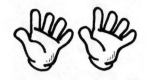

INGREDIENTS

1 (15-ounce) can yams (preferably water-packed)

1 (8-ounce) can crushed pineapple in juice

2 tablespoons apricot 100% fruit spread, melted

2 tablespoons walnuts, chopped

EQUIPMENT

Can opener

Knife

Cutting board

Small saucepan (or small bowl)

Measuring spoons

Large pan

Strainer

Potholders

Electric mixer

Serving dish

Spoon

DO THIS FIRST

▎ Check with an adult before you begin cooking and ask for help with the can opener, at the stove, and with the electric mixer.

▎ Read through the whole recipe and make sure you have all of the ingredients and equipment you need.

▎ Chop walnuts.

▎ Warm fruit spread in a small saucepan over low heat or in the microwave for about 20 seconds.

DIRECTIONS

1 Pour yams in a large pan (add water if there is very little liquid) and warm over medium heat.

2 When yams are hot, carefully drain off the liquid.

3 Using an electric mixer, mash yams until they are smooth.

4 Add pineapple and continue mixing 1–2 minutes until yams are thinner.

5 Spoon yams into a serving dish. Warm briefly in the microwave, if desired. Drizzle yams evenly with the melted apricot fruit spread and sprinkle with walnuts.

PREPARATION TIME
20 minutes

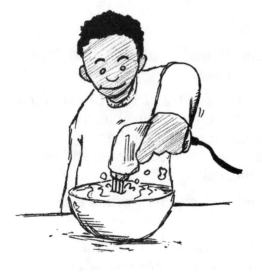

SERVES
4

SERVING SIZE
Heaping 1/2 cup

**Nutrition information
for 1 serving**

Calories	156
Total fat	3 g
Saturated fat	0 g
Cholesterol	0 mg
Sodium	13 mg
Total carbohydrate	33 g
Fiber	4 g
Protein	3 g

Exchanges

1 Starch
1 Fruit
1/2 Fat

Cheesy Zucchini Caterpillar

Z is for zucchini.

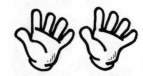

INGREDIENTS

1 straight zucchini (about 6 inches long)

1 teaspoon reduced-calorie margarine

1/8 teaspoon garlic salt

1/8 teaspoon onion powder

1 (3/4-ounce) slice fat-free processed sharp cheddar cheese, sliced in half

EQUIPMENT

Knife

Cutting board

Measuring spoons

Paper towels

Aluminum foil

Butter knife

Fork

Potholder

DO THIS FIRST

■ Check with an adult before you begin cooking and ask for help at the oven and with cutting.

■ Read through the whole recipe and make sure you have all of the ingredients and equipment you need.

■ Cut cheese slice in half.

DIRECTIONS

1 Preheat oven to 375°F.

2 Trim off ends of zucchini and throw them away.

3 About every 1/2 inch, slice 3/4 of the way through the zucchini, being careful not to cut all the way through (the slices should still be connected).

4 Gently dry zucchini with a paper towel.

5 Place zucchini on a piece of aluminum foil large enough to wrap around the zucchini.

6 Spread the top of the zucchini with margarine, then sprinkle evenly with garlic salt and onion powder.

7 Wrap the zucchini in foil and pinch foil closed.

8 Bake 30–35 minutes, or until zucchini is tender when poked with a fork.

9 Remove zucchini from the oven and carefully open the foil (watch out for steam).

10 Lay cheese slices down the length of the zucchini. Leave the foil open.

11 Place zucchini back in the oven 1–2 minutes, or until cheese is melted.

PREPARATION TIME
5 minutes

BAKING TIME
30–35 minutes

SERVINGS
1

SERVING SIZE
1 zucchini

Nutrition information for 1 serving

Calories	74
Total fat	2 g
Saturated fat	0 g
Cholesterol	3 mg
Sodium	466 mg
Total carbohydrate	8 g
Fiber	2 g
Protein	7 g

Exchanges

1 Meat, very lean
1 Vegetable
1/2 Fat

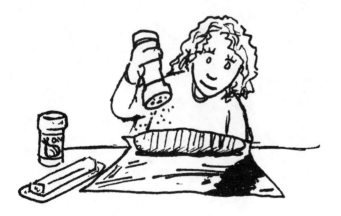

Recipe Section 2

Anytime in Between

Delicious treats that are terrific
after school, before sports,
or any other time of the day

Smiling Lion Face

A is for apple.

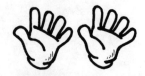

INGREDIENTS

- **2** tablespoons reduced-fat peanut butter
- **1** tablespoon + **1** teaspoon sweetened dried cranberries
- **1** small red unpeeled apple (about 4 ounces)
- **1** tablespoon lightly toasted rice cereal (such as Special K cereal)

EQUIPMENT

Apple corer (or paring knife)

Knife

Cutting board

Measuring spoons

Small mixing bowl

Butter knife (or spoon)

DO THIS FIRST

▌ Check with an adult before you begin cooking and ask for help with coring the apple and cutting.

▌ Read through the whole recipe and make sure you have all of the ingredients and equipment you need.

DIRECTIONS

1 Place peanut butter in a small bowl; set aside.

2 Lay aside 4 cranberries. Stir the rest into the peanut butter; set aside.

3 Using an apple corer or paring knife, carefully remove the apple core and seeds and throw them away. You should have about a 1 1/2-inch wide opening in the apple.

4 Using a butter knife or spoon, fill the center of the apple with the peanut butter mixture. Let the peanut butter spread slightly outside the opening in the apple.

5 Cut each of the 4 remaining cranberries in half. Make a smiley face on
top of the peanut butter using the
cranberry pieces: placing them cut
side down, use 2 for eyes, 1 for the
nose, and 5 for the smile.

6 Stick cereal around the edge of the
peanut butter to make the lion's
mane.

PREPARATION TIME
10 minutes

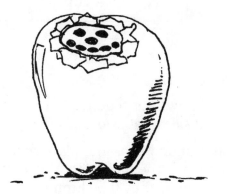

SERVINGS
1

SERVING SIZE
1 apple

**Nutrition information
for 1 serving**

Calories	281
Total fat	12 g
Saturated fat	2 g
Cholesterol	0 mg
Sodium	193 mg
Total carbohydrate	39 g
Fiber	6 g
Protein	9 g

Exchanges

2 1/2 Starch
1 Meat, high fat
1/2 Fat

Black Bean Flats

B is for black beans.

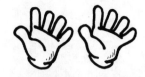

INGREDIENTS

1/2 cup light sour cream

2 tablespoons thick and chunky salsa

1 (15-ounce) can black beans

1 (10-ounce) can diced tomatoes and green chilies, undrained

1 teaspoon dried leaf oregano

1/4 teaspoon garlic powder

3/4 cup (3 ounces) finely shredded reduced-fat cheddar cheese, divided

9 (6-inch) corn tortillas

EQUIPMENT

Can opener

Grater (optional)

Measuring cups

Measuring spoons

Small mixing bowl

Strainer

Pan

Potato masher (or fork)

Long-handled mixing spoon

Plates

Spoon

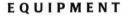

DIRECTIONS

1 In a small bowl, stir together sour cream and salsa; set aside.

2 Rinse and drain beans and place them in a pan. Mash them up with a potato masher or fork—they'll be lumpy.

3 Add diced tomatoes and green chilies, oregano, and garlic powder. Stir well. Bring to a boil over medium-high heat and cook uncovered for 20 minutes, or until thickened; stir occasionally.

4 Remove from heat and stir in 1/2 cup cheese.

5 Warm corn tortillas if you like according to the package directions.

6 Lay tortillas on plates or a flat serving tray. Lightly spread the sour cream mixture over each tortilla. Spoon a little less than 1/2 cup beans in the center of each tortilla (the beans will spread out). Using the remaining 1/4 cup cheese, put a few shreds of cheese on top in the center of the beans.

7 Let stand 5 minutes for cheese to melt and beans to thicken further.

PREPARATION TIME **35 minutes**   STANDING TIME **5 minutes**

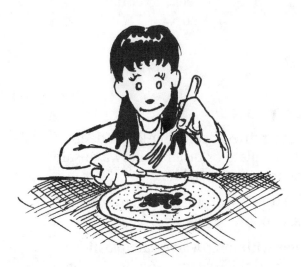

GOOD TO KNOW

▮ You can lower the fat content of the recipe further by using fat-free sour cream instead of light sour cream.

▮ These are a little messy, so eat them with a fork and knife.

SERVINGS
9

SERVING SIZE
1 bean flat

Nutrition information for 1 serving

Calories	148
Total fat	4 g
Saturated fat	2 g
Cholesterol	11 mg
Sodium	329 mg
Total carbohydrate	22 g
Fiber	4 g
Protein	8 g

Exchanges

1 1/2 Starch
1/2 Fat

Corny Fiesta Dip

C is for corn.

INGREDIENTS

1 (16-ounce) can fat-free refried beans

1 (8 3/4-ounce) can no-salt-added corn, drained well

1 (12-ounce) jar thick and chunky mild salsa

1 cup (4 ounces) finely shredded reduced-fat cheddar cheese

EQUIPMENT

Can opener

Strainer

Grater (optional)

Measuring cups

Microwave-safe dish

Potholders

Large mixing bowl

Long-handled mixing spoon

Microwave-safe plastic wrap

DO THIS FIRST

- Check with an adult before you begin cooking and ask for help with using the can opener, grater, and at the microwave.

- Read through the whole recipe and make sure you have all of the ingredients and equipment you need.

- Open corn and drain well.

- If not using pre-packaged shredded cheese, grate enough reduced-fat cheddar cheese to equal 1 cup.

DIRECTIONS

1 Spread refried beans in a glass deep-dish pie plate or other microwave-safe serving dish; set aside.

2 In a large bowl, stir together corn and salsa. Spoon evenly over beans.

3 Cover with microwave-safe plastic wrap and microwave 5-6 minutes on HIGH, or until bubbly.

4 Carefully pull back plastic wrap (watch out for steam) and sprinkle cheese over the top of the dip.

5 Cover dip again with plastic wrap and let stand 5 minutes, or until cheese is melted.

6 Serve with baked tortilla chips.

PREPARATION TIME
20 minutes

▮ You can do steps 1 and 2 up to 2 days ahead of serving time, then cover and refrigerate dip.

▮ Leftover dip tastes great when re-heated.

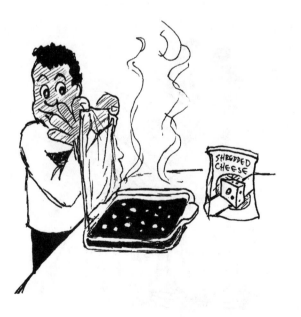

SERVINGS
16

SERVING SIZE
1/4 cup

Nutrition information for 1 serving

Calories	57
Total fat	2 g
Saturated fat	1 g
Cholesterol	5 mg
Sodium	326 mg
Total carbohydrate	8 g
Fiber	2 g
Protein	4 g

Exchanges

1/2 Starch

Camp Kids Crunch

D is for dried fruit and the diabetes camp kids who taste-tested this recipe.

INGREDIENTS

2 1/2 cups crispy corn puff cereal (such as Kix cereal)

2 1/2 cups frosted oat cereal with marshmallows (such as Lucky Charms cereal)

1 1/4 cups pretzel fish (such as Pepperidge Farm Pretzel Fish)

1 1/4 cups mixed dried fruit

3/4 cup salted soy nuts

3/4 cup fruit flavored bite-sized candy (such as Skittles)

EQUIPMENT

Measuring cups

Airtight container

DO THIS FIRST

▮ Check with an adult before you begin cooking.

▮ Read through the whole recipe and make sure you have all of the ingredients and equipment you need.

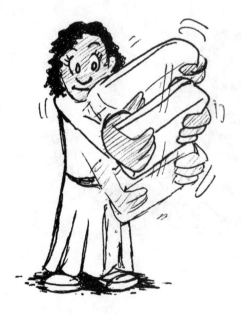

DIRECTIONS

1 Combine all ingredients in an air-tight container.

2 Put on lid and seal tightly.

3 Shake to combine.

PREPARATION TIME
10 minutes

SERVINGS
18

SERVING SIZE
1/2 cup

Nutrition information for 1 serving

Calories	142
Total fat	2 g
Saturated fat	0 g
Cholesterol	0 mg
Sodium	177 mg
Total carbohydrate	27 g
Fiber	2 g
Protein	4 g

Exchanges

2 Starch

"Egg"cellent Eggplant Sticks

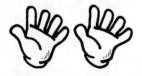

E is for eggplant.

INGREDIENTS

butter-flavored cooking spray

1/4 cup + **2** tablespoons dry bread crumbs

3 tablespoons grated Parmesan cheese

1/8 teaspoon garlic powder

3/4 teaspoon Italian seasoning

2 egg whites

2 teaspoons water

1 small eggplant (about 1 pound)

1 1/2 cups spaghetti sauce

EQUIPMENT

Knife

Cutting board

Measuring cups

Measuring spoons

Baking sheet

2 shallow dishes

Long-handled mixing spoon

Whisk

Pan

Potholder

Serving dish

DO THIS FIRST

▌ Check with an adult before you begin cooking and ask for help at the oven, with the cutting, and at the stove/microwave.

▌ Read through the whole recipe and make sure you have all of the ingredients and equipment you need.

DIRECTIONS

1 Preheat oven to 400°F.

2 Spray a baking sheet with cooking spray; set aside.

3 In a shallow dish (such as a pie pan), combine bread crumbs, Parmesan cheese, garlic powder, and Italian seasoning; stir well and set aside.

4 In another shallow dish, combine egg whites and water; beat with a whisk until frothy; set aside.

5 Trim ends off the eggplant. Cut eggplant into 4 pieces lengthwise, then cut each into sticks about 1/2 inch wide and 3 inches long.

6 Roll each eggplant stick in crumb mixture, then dip in egg white, then roll in crumb mixture again to coat.

7 Place crumb-coated eggplant sticks on the baking sheet and spray each well with cooking spray.

8 Bake 15–18 minutes, or until golden brown and tender.

9 Meanwhile, warm spaghetti sauce.

10 Remove baked eggplant sticks from the baking sheet to a serving dish and serve with warm spaghetti sauce.

PREPARATION TIME
30 minutes

BAKING TIME
15–18 minutes

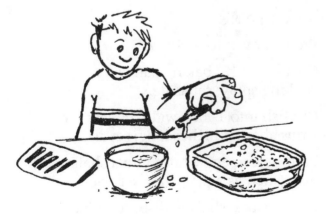

GOOD TO KNOW
Try serving with ketchup instead of spaghetti sauce.

SERVINGS
8

SERVING SIZE
1/8 of the eggplant sticks with dipping sauce

Nutrition information for 1 serving

Calories	100
Total fat	3 g
Saturated fat	1 g
Cholesterol	3 mg
Sodium	338 mg
Total carbohydrate	15 g
Fiber	3 g
Protein	4 g

Exchanges

1 Starch
1/2 Fat

Flaky Fish Fingers

F is for fish.

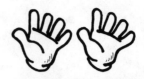

INGREDIENTS

butter-flavored cooking spray

1 8-ounce white fish fillet (about 1/4-inch thick)

2 egg whites, beaten

1/8 teaspoon salt

1/8 teaspoon lemon pepper seasoning

1/8 teaspoon garlic powder

1 teaspoon grated Parmesan cheese

1/4 cup + **1** tablespoon prepackaged dry bread crumbs

EQUIPMENT

Whisk (or electric mixer, or fork)

Small mixing bowl

Measuring spoons

Measuring cups

Knife

Cutting board

9″ x 13″ baking pan

2 shallow dishes (pie plate)

Long-handled mixing spoon

Potholder

DO THIS FIRST

▌ Check with an adult before you begin cooking and ask for help at the oven and with cutting.

▌ Read through the whole recipe and make sure you have all of the ingredients and equipment you need.

▌ Beat 2 egg whites.

DIRECTIONS

1 Preheat oven to 425°F.

2 Coat a 9″ x 13″ baking pan with cooking spray; set aside.

3 Cut fish into 1-inch wide "fingers" or strips about 4 inches long; set aside.

4 Pour beaten egg whites into a shallow dish (such as a pie plate); set aside.

5 In a separate shallow dish, combine salt, lemon pepper seasoning, garlic powder, Parmesan cheese, and bread crumbs; stir well with a spoon, then set aside.

6 Dip each fish "finger" into egg whites, then into bread crumb mixture, turning over to coat well; shake off extra crumbs back into the dish. Place fish on the pan. Continue until all fish "fingers" are coated with crumbs.

7 Spray fish evenly with butter-flavored cooking spray.

8 Bake for 10–12 minutes (thicker "fingers" may take longer), or until fish flakes easily with a fork. Be careful not to overbake. After taking the pan out of the oven, let the fish stand 2–3 minutes before moving it to a serving plate.

PREPARATION TIME
15 minutes

BAKING TIME
10–12 minutes

STANDING TIME
2–3 minutes

SERVINGS
4

SERVING SIZE
2 ounces (about 3 fingers)

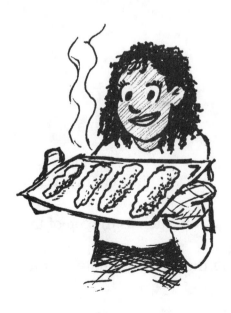

**Nutrition information
for 1 serving**

Calories	96
Total fat	1 g
Saturated fat	0 g
Cholesterol	30 mg
Sodium	244 mg
Total carbohydrate	6 g
Fiber	0 g
Protein	14 g

Exchanges

1/2 Starch
2 Meat, very lean

Grow A Windowsill Herb Garden!

G is for garden.

WHAT YOU'LL NEED

- An empty cardboard egg carton with lid
- Potting soil
- Seeds from your favorite herbs (basil, marjoram, oregano, parsley and thyme work well)

WHAT YOU'LL DO

1 Fill each egg hole with potting soil.
2 Put two seeds from your favorite herb in each hole.

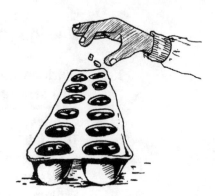

3 Cover the seeds with a small amount of dirt. Add just enough water to moisten.
4 Close the carton and place somewhere warm, such as the top of the refrigerator.
5 Check the seeds every day to make sure the dirt stays moist, but not overly wet.

6 When you see sprouts from the tiny plants, move the egg carton to a sunny spot. Close the lid at night.

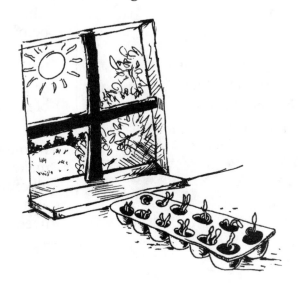

7 When the seedlings are an inch high, fertilize them with a water-soluble plant food.

8 When the seedlings grow a bit bigger, plant each section of the egg carton in a pot or in your garden.

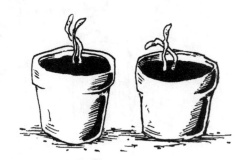

9 You can harvest your herbs by taking leaves off the top to add to your cooking. If you dry the leaves in the fall, you can use them all winter!

PB&J Hummus

H is for hummus.

INGREDIENTS

3/4 cup canned garbanzo beans
1/4 cup reduced-fat peanut butter
1/4 cup unsweetened apple juice
1/4 teaspoon ground cinnamon
1/4 cup blueberry 100% fruit spread

EQUIPMENT

Can opener
Blender
Measuring cups
Measuring spoons
Strainer
Rubber spatula
Spoon
Serving bowl

DO THIS FIRST

▌ Check with an adult before you begin cooking and ask for help with using the can opener and blender.

▌ Read through the whole recipe and make sure you have all of the ingredients and equipment you need.

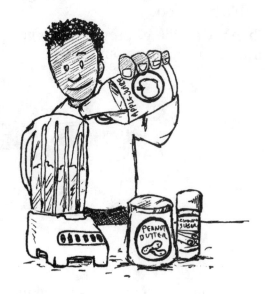

DIRECTIONS

1 Rinse and drain garbanzo beans. Pour them into the blender.

2 Add peanut butter, apple juice, and cinnamon to the blender; scrape down sides of blender with a rubber spatula if needed. Cover and blend until smooth.

3 Spoon hummus into a bowl and spoon a layer of fruit spread over the top.

PREPARATION TIME
10 minutes

GOOD TO KNOW

▌ You can use other flavors of fruit spread or leave it off all together.

▌ Try serving hummus with crackers, graham crackers, banana chunks, or celery sticks.

SERVES
8

SERVING SIZE
2 tablespoons

**Nutrition information
for 1 serving**

Calories 94
Total fat . . . . 3 g
   Saturated fat . . . . 1 g
Cholesterol . . . . 0 mg
Sodium . . . . 70 mg
Total carbohydrate . . . . . 14 g
   Fiber . . . . 2 g
Protein . . . . 3 g

Exchanges

1/2 Starch
1/2 Fruit
1/2 Fat

Brown Bear Cups

I is for ice cream.

INGREDIENTS

3 maraschino cherries

2 cups fat-free no sugar added chocolate ice cream

1 (4-ounce) package single-serving graham cracker crusts

12 chocolate wafer cookies

12 milk chocolate chips

EQUIPMENT

Knife

Cutting board

Measuring cups

Paper towel

Ice cream scoop

Airtight container (optional)

DO THIS FIRST

▌ Check with an adult before you begin cooking and ask for help with slicing.

▌ Read through the whole recipe and make sure you have all of the ingredients and equipment you need.

DIRECTIONS

1 Rinse maraschino cherries, slice each in half, and set upside down on a paper towel to drain well.

2 Place 1 rounded scoop (about 1/3 cup) ice cream into each crust.

3 Stick 1 chocolate wafer cookie into each side of the ice cream scoops for ears.

4 Press 2 chocolate chips into each ice cream scoop for eyes.

5 Press 1 maraschino cherry half onto each ice cream scoop for a nose.

6 Eat right away or seal tightly in an airtight container and freeze.

PREPARATION TIME
15 minutes

GOOD TO KNOW

These store well in the freezer so you can make them ahead of time for a party.

SERVINGS
6

SERVING SIZE
1 bear cup

**Nutrition information
for 1 serving**

Calories. 243	
Total fat. . . . . 7 g	
Saturated fat . . . . 2 g	
Cholesterol. . . . . 0 mg	
Sodium . . . . 249 mg	
Total carbohydrate. . . . . 38 g	
Fiber . . . . 1 g	
Protein. . . . . 4 g	

Exchanges

2 1/2 Other carbohydrate
1 1/2 Fat

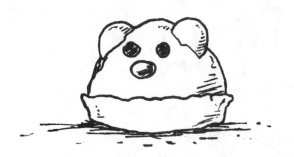

Jicama Shoestrings

J is for jicama.

INGREDIENTS

1 1/2 pounds (or 24 ounces) jicama
(Mexican potato)

1/4 teaspoon salt

1 tablespoon fresh-squeezed
lemon juice

EQUIPMENT

Knife

Cutting board

Measuring spoons

Paper towel

Airtight container

DO THIS FIRST

▌ Check with an adult
before you begin
cooking and ask for
help with peeling
and slicing.

▌ Read through the
whole recipe and
make sure you have
all of the ingredients
and equipment you
need.

▌ Squeeze 1 tablespoon
juice from a fresh
lemon.

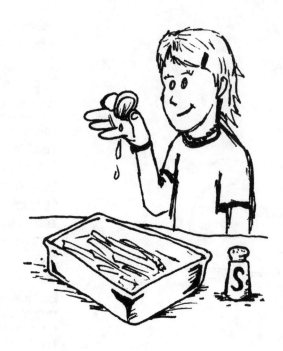

DIRECTIONS

1 Rinse jicama and dry with a paper towel.

2 Cut the tough peel from the jicama.

3 Cut the jicama into sticks or shoe-strings (about 2 1/2 inches long and 1/4 inch wide).

4 Place the jicama sticks in an airtight container. Sprinkle with salt and drizzle with lemon juice.

5 Place lid tightly on the container and shake it 15 times.

6 Refrigerate leftovers.

PREPARATION TIME
15 minutes

SERVINGS
12

SERVING SIZE
1/2 cup jicama shoestrings

Nutrition information for 1 serving

Calories 20
Total fat . . . . 0 g
  Saturated fat . . . . 0 g
Cholesterol . . . . 0 mg
Sodium . . . . 51 mg
Total carbohydrate . . . . . . 5 g
  Fiber . . . . 3 g
Protein . . . . 0 g

Exchanges

1 Vegetable

Fun Fizz

K is for Kool-Aid.

INGREDIENTS

1 (0.3-ounce) package artificially-sweetened cherry-flavored Kool-Aid drink mix

1 (0.45-ounce) package artificially-sweetened lemonade-flavored Kool-Aid drink mix

4 quarts cold water, divided

1 (2-liter) bottle diet lemon-lime soda

EQUIPMENT

Measuring cups

2 pitchers

Long-handled mixing spoon

Ice cube trays

Pitcher (or punch bowl)

DO THIS FIRST
▌ Check with an adult before you begin cooking.
▌ Read through the whole recipe and make sure you have all of the ingredients and equipment you need.

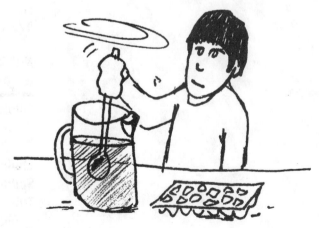

DIRECTIONS

1 Pour each package of Kool-Aid mix into a separate pitcher. Add 2 quarts cold water to each pitcher. Stir until Kool-Aid dissolves.

2 Carefully pour Kool-Aid into ice cube trays (about 2 tablespoons per cube) and freeze until solid (about 3 hours).

3 Place Kool-Aid cubes in a punch bowl or pitcher and add diet lemon-lime soda. For a single serving, place 3 cubes of each flavor Kool-Aid in a tall glass and add 3/4 cup (6 ounces) diet lemon-lime soda.

4 Serve right away.

PREPARATION TIME	FREEZING TIME
15 minutes	**3 hours**

SERVINGS
10

SERVING SIZE
1/10 of recipe

Nutrition information for 1 serving

Calories 8
Total fat . . . . 0 g
   Saturated fat . . . . 0 g
Cholesterol . . . . 0 mg
Sodium . . . . 24 mg
Total carbohydrate . . . . . . 2 g
   Fiber . . . . 0 g
Protein . . . . 0 g

Exchanges

Free food

Chef Salad Roll-ups

L is for lettuce.

INGREDIENTS

1 large leaf green leaf lettuce

1 (1-ounce) slice lean deli ham

1 (1-ounce) slice deli turkey breast

1 tablespoon shredded carrot

1 tablespoon shredded reduced-fat cheddar cheese

2 tablespoons alfalfa sprouts

low-fat dressing (optional)

EQUIPMENT

Grater (optional)

Measuring spoons

Plastic wrap (optional)

DO THIS FIRST

▌ Check with an adult before you begin cooking and ask for help with the grater.

▌ Read through the whole recipe and make sure you have all of the ingredients and equipment you need.

▌ If not using pre-packaged shredded cheese, grate enough reduced-fat cheddar cheese to make 1 tablespoon.

▌ If not using pre-packaged shredded carrot, grate enough carrot to make 1 tablespoon.

DIRECTIONS

1 Lay lettuce leaf on the counter. Top it with the ham, then turkey. Sprinkle on shredded carrot and cheese. Put sprouts on top.

2 Roll up like a jellyroll.

3 If you are not eating the roll-up right away, wrap it in plastic wrap and chill.

4 Eat plain or dip in low-fat dressing.

PREPARATION TIME
5 minutes

SERVINGS
1

SERVING SIZE
1 roll-up

Nutrition information for 1 serving

Calories	98
Total fat	4 g
Saturated fat	2 g
Cholesterol	34 mg
Sodium	679 mg
Total carbohydrate	1 g
Fiber	0 g
Protein	15 g

Exchanges

2 Meat, lean

Mango Pops

M is for mango.

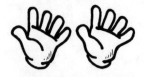

INGREDIENTS

- **1** (26-ounce) jar sliced mango in juice, drained
- **1** (8-ounce) container fat-free, artificially-sweetened vanilla-flavored yogurt
- **1/4** teaspoon lemon juice
- **1/4** teaspoon almond (or vanilla) extract

EQUIPMENT

Blender

Knife

Measuring spoons

6 (5-ounce) wax-coated paper cups

Aluminum foil

6 wooden craft (popsicle) sticks

DO THIS FIRST

- Check with an adult before you begin cooking and ask for help using the blender and knife.
- Read through the whole recipe and make sure you have all of the ingredients and equipment you need.

DIRECTIONS

1 Place mango, yogurt, lemon juice, and extract in a blender and cover tightly with lid. Blend until smooth.

2 Pour mango mixture into each of 6 wax-coated paper cups, filling 3/4 full.

3 Cover the top of each cup with foil.

4 Using a pointed knife, carefully poke a small slit in the middle of the foil over each cup and insert a wooden popsicle stick into mango mixture in the cup.

5 Freeze until firm (about 6 hours).

6 Tear paper cup off pop to eat.

PREPARATION TIME
15 minutes

FREEZING TIME
6 hours

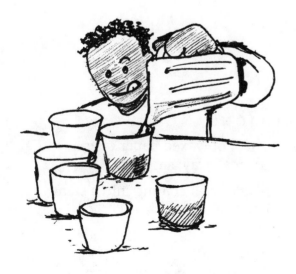

SERVINGS
6

SERVING SIZE
1 pop

**Nutrition information
for 1 serving**

Calories	74
Total fat	0 g
Saturated fat	0 g
Cholesterol	1 mg
Sodium	29 mg
Total carbohydrate	17 g
Fiber	1 g
Protein	1 g

Exchanges

1 Fruit

Chocolate-Dunked Nilla Wafers

N is for Nilla Wafer.

INGREDIENTS

8 Rainbow Nilla Wafers

1 tablespoon chocolate Magic Shell topping

1/4 teaspoon nonpareil sprinkles

EQUIPMENT

Measuring spoons

Waxed paper

Plate (or small tray)

Cup (or deep bowl)

Airtight container

DO THIS FIRST

▌ Check with an adult before you begin cooking.

▌ Read through the whole recipe and make sure you have all of the ingredients and equipment you need.

DIRECTIONS

1 Lay a sheet of waxed paper over a plate or small tray; set aside.

2 Pour Magic Shell coating into a small, deep bowl or cup.

3 Dunk a Nilla Wafer into the chocolate, coating half the cookie. Sprinkle chocolate-coated portion with nonpareil sprinkles. Lay cookie on waxed paper. Repeat with remaining cookies.

4 Refrigerate cookies, uncovered, for 20 minutes, or until chocolate hardens.

5 Store in an airtight container in the refrigerator.

PREPARATION TIME
5 minutes

CHILLING TIME
20 minutes

GOOD TO KNOW

You can also use plain Nilla Wafers in place of Rainbow Nilla Wafers.

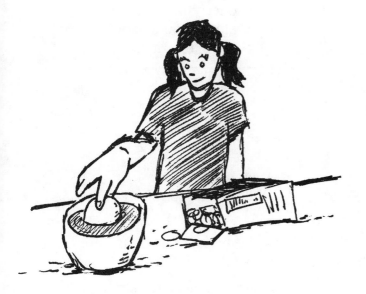

SERVINGS
2

SERVING SIZE
4 cookies

**Nutrition information
for 1 serving**

Calories	125
Total fat	7 g
Saturated fat	3 g
Cholesterol	8 mg
Sodium	61 mg
Total carbohydrate	16 g
Fiber	1 g
Protein	1 g

Exchanges

1 Starch
1 Fat

SunShine Salad

O is for orange.

INGREDIENTS

- **1** (11-ounce) can mandarin oranges in juice, drained
- **1** (20-ounce) can pineapple chunks in juice, drained
- **1** (15-ounce) can sliced peaches in juice, drained
- **2** large bananas (about 8 ounces each), sliced
- **14** maraschino cherries, cut into quarters and drained
- **1** (1-ounce) box fat-free artificially-sweetened vanilla-flavored instant pudding mix
- **1** cup unsweetened orange juice

EQUIPMENT

Can opener

Knife

Cutting board

Measuring cups

2 large bowls

Whisk

Long-handled mixing spoon

DO THIS FIRST

- ▌Check with an adult before you begin cooking and ask for help with the can opener and knife.
- ▌Read through the whole recipe and make sure you have all of the ingredients and equipment you need.
- ▌Open the cans of fruit and drain off the juice.
- ▌Slice the bananas.
- ▌Cut each maraschino cherry into 4 pieces and lay on a paper towel to drain.

DIRECTIONS

1 Place mandarin oranges, pineapple chunks, peaches, banana slices, and maraschino cherry pieces in a large bowl; set aside.

2 In another bowl, combine pudding mix and orange juice; mix using a wire whisk. Pour over fruit. Stir well so that fruit is coated with pudding.

3 Chill 30 minutes.

PREPARATION TIME
15 minutes

CHILLING TIME
30 minutes

GOOD TO KNOW

If making this salad several hours ahead (or a day or two ahead), wait and add the banana right before serving.

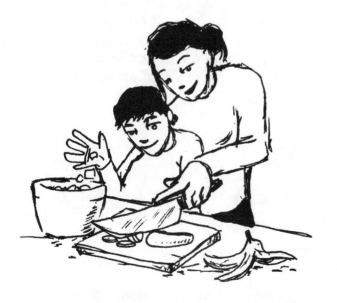

SERVINGS
13

SERVING SIZE
1/2 cup

**Nutrition information
for 1 serving**

Calories	78
Total fat	0 g
Saturated fat	0 g
Cholesterol	0 mg
Sodium	104 mg
Total carbohydrate	19 g
Fiber	1 g
Protein	1 g

Exchanges

1 1/2 Fruit

Pizza Face

P is for pizza.

INGREDIENTS

1/2 English muffin

1 tablespoon pizza sauce

2 olive slices (black or green)

1/2 cherry tomato

1 sliver green pepper

2 pieces pepperoni

1 tablespoon finely shredded part-skim mozzarella cheese

EQUIPMENT

Knife

Cutting board

Grater (optional)

Measuring spoons

Toaster

Baking sheet

Potholders

DO THIS FIRST

▌ Check with an adult before you begin cooking and ask for help at the oven, and with cutting and grater.

▌ Read through the whole recipe and make sure you have all of the ingredients and equipment you need.

▌ Cut olive slices, cherry tomato, and green pepper.

▌ If not using pre-packaged shredded mozzarella cheese, grate enough part-skim mozzarella to make 1 tablespoon.

DIRECTIONS

1 Preheat oven to 350°F.

2 Toast English muffin lightly in a toaster.

3 Lay English muffin on a baking sheet and spread pizza sauce over the top.

4 Make eyes with the olive slices.

5 Make a nose with the cherry tomato half.

6 Make a mouth with the green pepper.

7 Make ears with the pieces of pepperoni by laying them in the pizza sauce near the edge of the English muffin.

8 Make hair with the cheese.

9 Bake for 8–10 minutes, or until the cheese is melted and the pizza is heated through.

PREPARATION TIME
10 minutes

BAKING TIME
8–10 minutes

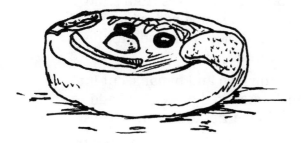

GOOD TO KNOW

This tastes best served right from the oven.

SERVES
1

SERVING SIZE
1 pizza

**Nutrition information
for 1 serving**

Calories	119
Total fat	4 g
Saturated fat	2 g
Cholesterol	7 mg
Sodium	387 mg
Total carbohydrate	15 g
Fiber	1 g
Protein	5 g

Exchanges

1 Starch
1 Fat

Fruit-Filled Quesadillas

Q is for quesadillas.

INGREDIENTS

Fruit salsa

1 cup fresh blueberries

1 cup fresh whole strawberries

1 kiwi fruit

1 small banana (about 4 ounces)

1 medium fresh peach (about 6 ounces)

2 tablespoons unsweetened orange juice

Filling

1/2 cup + **2** tablespoons reduced-fat spreadable cream cheese

1/4 cup + **1** tablespoon raspberry 100% fruit spread

Tortillas

1 teaspoon cinnamon

1 teaspoon nutmeg

1 tablespoon sugar butter-flavored cooking spray

10 (6-inch) flour tortillas

EQUIPMENT

Knife

Cutting board

Measuring spoons

Measuring cups

Large bowls

2 medium bowls

Plastic wrap

Nonstick skillet

Serving tray

Spoon

Pizza cutter (optional)

DIRECTIONS

1 Place blueberries in a large bowl; set aside.

2 Remove green leaves from strawberries, cut strawberries into small bite-sized pieces, and add to the blueberries.

3 Peel the kiwi and banana, cut into small bite-sized pieces, and add to the blueberries and strawberries.

4 Peel the peach and remove the pit. Cut the peach into small bite-sized pieces and add to the other fruits.

5 Evenly pour orange juice over the fruit and toss to coat. Cover and chill slightly in the refrigerator.

6 In a separate bowl, stir together cream cheese and fruit spread until well mixed; set aside.

7 Combine cinnamon, nutmeg, and sugar in a bowl and stir well; set aside.

8 Spray the top and bottom of each tortilla with cooking spray. Place tortillas in a nonstick skillet and warm them over medium heat (about 1–2 minutes) until they begin to puff up. Turn tortillas over and continue cooking until puffed and golden (about 1–2 minutes more). Sprinkle the top lightly with the sugar/spice mixture and remove from the pan to a plate.

9 On a large serving tray, place 5 tortillas, spice side down. Spread 1/5 of the cream cheese (about 3 tablespoons) mixture evenly over each tortilla. Then spread 2/3 cup fruit over the cream cheese. Top with a second tortilla, spice side up.

10 Cut each quesadilla into 4 equal pieces (a pizza cutter makes cutting easy).

11 Serve right away.

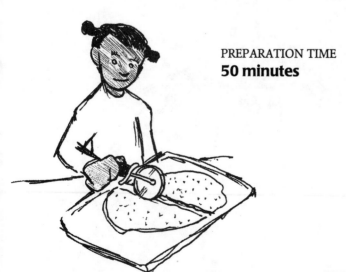

PREPARATION TIME
50 minutes

GOOD TO KNOW

This is yummy but messy, so eat with a fork and knife or have lots of napkins on hand.

SERVES
10

SERVING SIZE
2 pieces or 1/2 quesadilla

**Nutrition information
for 1 serving**

Calories	193
Total fat	5 g
Saturated fat	3 g
Cholesterol	10 mg
Sodium	209 mg
Total carbohydrate	32 g
Fiber	3 g
Protein	5 g

Exchanges

1 Starch
1 Fruit
1 Fat

Roast Beef Roll-up

R is for roast beef.

INGREDIENTS

1 (6-inch) flour tortilla

2 teaspoons steak sauce (such as A-1 steak sauce)

2 ounces lean deli roast beef, thinly sliced

1 (1-ounce) stick string cheese

EQUIPMENT

Measuring spoons

Pastry brush (or spoon, or butter knife)

Toothpicks

DO THIS FIRST

▌ Check with an adult before you begin cooking.

▌ Read through the whole recipe and make sure you have all of the ingredients and equipment you need.

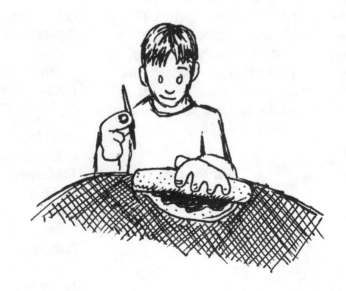

DIRECTIONS

1 Lay flour tortilla on the counter.

2 Pour steak sauce into the center of the flour tortilla and spread evenly over the tortilla with a pastry brush, the back of a spoon, or a dull knife.

3 Lay roast beef slices evenly over the tortilla.

4 Place the stick of string cheese on one side of the tortilla, then roll tortilla and meat around it. Stick a toothpick in each end to hold the roll-up together.

PREPARATION TIME
5 minutes

If you want to, heat the roll-up for 20–30 seconds in the microwave. Be sure to ask an adult for help.

SERVINGS
1

SERVING SIZE
1 roll-up

**Nutrition information
for 1 serving**

Calories	280
Total fat	10 g
Saturated fat	5 g
Cholesterol	54 mg
Sodium	827 mg
Total carbohydrate	19 g
Fiber	1 g
Protein	25 g

Exchanges

1 1/2 Starch
3 Meat, lean

upSide-Down Pizza Soup

S is for soup.

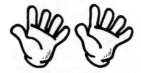

INGREDIENTS

1 pound (16 ounces) ground sirloin

1 (14-ounce) can fat-free beef broth

2 (14 1/2-ounce) cans diced tomatoes seasoned with basil, garlic, and oregano, undrained

1 (6-ounce) can tomato paste

1 small onion, chopped

1 (4-ounce) can sliced mushrooms, drained

35 croutons (1 3/4 ounces total)

3/4 cup + **2** tablespoons shredded part-skim mozzarella cheese (about 3 1/2 ounces)

EQUIPMENT

Can opener

Knife

Cutting board

Grater (optional)

Measuring cups

Measuring spoons

Nonstick skillet

Large pan (or stockpot) with lid

Long-handled mixing spoon

Bowls

DO THIS FIRST

▌ Check with an adult before you begin cooking and ask for help at the stove, with the can opener, cutting, and with the grater.

▌ Read through the whole recipe and make sure you have all of the ingredients and equipment you need.

▌ Chop 1 small onion.

▌ Open mushrooms and drain.

▌ If not using pre-packaged shredded mozzarella cheese, grate enough part-skim mozzarella to make 3/4 cup + 2 tablespoons.

DIRECTIONS

1 Brown ground sirloin in a nonstick skillet over medium-high heat until no longer pink (about 5–6 minutes). Drain well.

2 In a large pan or stockpot, combine browned meat, beef broth, tomatoes, tomato paste, chopped onion, and mushrooms. Stir well. Cover the pan with a lid and bring to a boil over high heat. Reduce the heat to medium and simmer for 30 minutes; frequently remove the lid and stir— watch out for steam.

3 Spoon 1 cup soup into each bowl and top with 5 croutons and 2 tablespoons cheese.

PREPARATION TIME
15 minutes

COOKING TIME
30 minutes

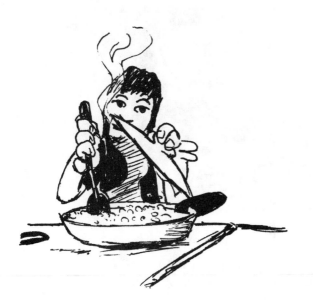

SERVINGS
7

SERVING SIZE
1 cup

Nutrition information for 1 serving

Calories	238
Total fat	6 g
Saturated fat	3 g
Cholesterol	51 mg
Sodium	1084 mg
Total carbohydrate	22 g
Fiber	2 g
Protein	23 g

Exchanges

1/2 Starch
3 Vegetable
2 Meat, lean

Tiny Stuffed Tomato Poppers

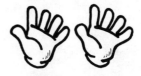

T is for tomato.

INGREDIENTS

1/4 cup fat-free spreadable cream cheese

1/4 cup + **1** tablespoon light pasteurized
processed cheese spread (such as
Cheez Whiz Light)

1/2 teaspoon dried chopped chives

1 ounce lean deli ham, finely chopped

30 cherry tomatoes

EQUIPMENT

Knife
Cutting board
Measuring cups
Measuring spoons
Medium mixing bowl
Rubber spatula
Spoon
Plastic wrap

DO THIS FIRST

▎ Check with an adult
before you begin
cooking and ask for
help with cutting.

▎ Read through the
whole recipe and
make sure you have
all of the ingredients
and equipment you
need.

▎ Finely chop the ham.

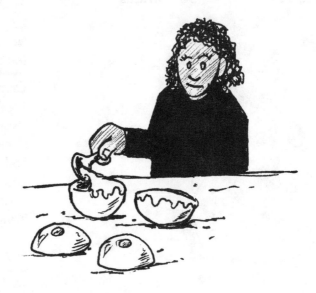

DIRECTIONS

1 Put cream cheese, cheese spread, and chives in a bowl and mix together using a rubber spatula.

2 Add ham and stir until well mixed; set aside.

3 Remove green leaves from tomatoes. Cut each tomato in half crosswise (from side to side). Spread bottom halves of tomatoes with 1 teaspoon cheese mixture. Top with top halves of the tomatoes.

4 Cover and refrigerate until serving time.

PREPARATION TIME
25 minutes

SERVINGS
10

SERVING SIZE
3 tomatoes

**Nutrition information
for 1 serving**

Calories	41
Total fat	1 g
Saturated fat	1 g
Cholesterol	7 mg
Sodium	203 mg
Total carbohydrate	4 g
Fiber	1 g
Protein	3 g

Exchanges

1 Vegetable

Chocolate-Baked Ugli Fruit

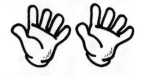

U is for Ugli fruit.

INGREDIENTS

1 Ugli fruit at room temperature

1 tablespoon mini semisweet chocolate chips

1 tablespoon raspberry 100% fruit spread

EQUIPMENT

Knife

Cutting board

Measuring spoons

Spoon

Baking pan

Potholder

Small microwave-safe bowl

Small saucepan (optional)

DO THIS FIRST

▌ Check with an adult before you begin cooking and ask for help with the oven, with cutting, and at the microwave.

▌ Read through the whole recipe and make sure you have all of the ingredients and equipment you need.

DIRECTIONS

1 Preheat oven to 350°F.

2 Cut a thin slice off each end of the Ugli fruit, then slice the Ugli fruit in half crosswise.

3 Using a knife, gently cut around Ugli fruit sections to loosen them inside the skin; remove any seeds.

4 Sprinkle each Ugli fruit half with 1/2 tablespoon chocolate chips.

5 Place in a pan and bake uncovered for 5–7 minutes, or until chocolate chips soften.

6 Place the fruit spread in a small microwave-safe bowl and heat for 20–30 seconds, or until runny (or warm it in a small saucepan on the stove over low-medium heat).

7 Use a spoon to drizzle the fruit spread over each Ugli fruit half and into the centers.

8 Serve warm.

PREPARATION TIME
10 minutes

BAKING TIME
5–7 minutes

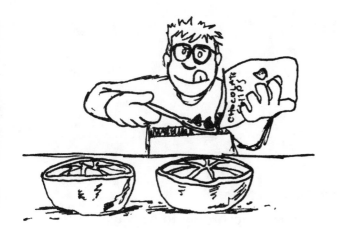

SERVES
2

SERVING SIZE
1/2 Ugli fruit

Nutrition information for 1 serving

Calories	105
Total fat	2 g
Saturated fat	1 g
Cholesterol	0 mg
Sodium	3 mg
Total carbohydrate	21 g
Fiber	3 g
Protein	1 g

Exchanges

1 1/2 Fruit

Sensational Overnight Vegetable Salad

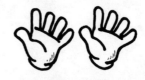

V is for vegetable salad.

INGREDIENTS

2 ounces uncooked bow tie pasta
(just over 3/4 cup)

1 cup broccoli florets

1 cup cauliflower florets

1/2 cup carrot slices

1/2 cup grape tomatoes (cherry tomatoes
can be substituted)

1/2 cup light Italian dressing

EQUIPMENT

Knife

Cutting board

Measuring cups

Pan

Potholder

Long-handled mixing spoon

Strainer

Serving dish

Plastic wrap

DO THIS FIRST

▋ Check with an adult before you begin cooking and ask for help with cutting.

▋ Read through the whole recipe and make sure you have all of the ingredients and equipment you need.

▋ Cut enough bite-sized pieces of broccoli tops and cauliflower tops to make 1 cup of each.

▋ Cut enough bite-sized slices of carrot to make 1/2 cup.

DIRECTIONS

1 Cook pasta according to package directions, omitting any salt. Carefully drain well, rinse in cold water, and drain well again. Pour into a serving dish.

2 Add broccoli, cauliflower, carrots, and tomatoes to the pasta. Drizzle dressing over top, then toss to coat well. Cover and refrigerate 6–8 hours, or overnight.

3 Before serving, toss well.

PREPARATION TIME
25 minutes

CHILLING TIME
6–8 hours

▌ Avoid cutting up the vegetables by using broccoli, cauliflower, and carrots purchased from a salad bar or prepackaged in bags ready for use.

▌ If choking is a concern, cut each tomato into 4 pieces.

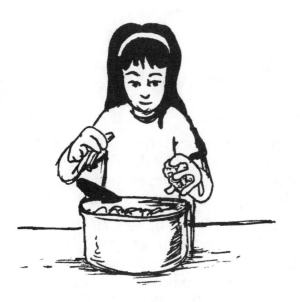

SERVES
8

SERVING SIZE
1/2 cup

**Nutrition information
for 1 serving**

Calories	64
Total fat	2 g
Saturated fat	0 g
Cholesterol	0 mg
Sodium	124 mg
Total carbohydrate	9 g
Fiber	1 g
Protein	2 g

Exchanges

1/2 Starch
1/2 Fat

watercolor Toast

W is for whole-wheat.

INGREDIENTS

1/2 cup water
  red food coloring
  yellow food coloring
  blue food coloring
  green food coloring
2 slices whole-wheat bread

EQUIPMENT

Measuring spoons
Toaster
4 small bowls
4 spoons
Pastry brush (or new
  paintbrush)

DO THIS FIRST

▮ Check with an adult before you begin cooking and ask for help with the toaster.

▮ Read through the whole recipe and make sure you have all of the ingredients and equipment you need.

DIRECTIONS

1 Pour 2 tablespoons water into each of 4 small bowls. Add 3 drops of one food coloring to each bowl of water; use a separate spoon to stir each well.

2 Use a pastry brush or new, clean paintbrush to "paint" designs on the bread using the watercolors. Each time you dip the brush in a water-color, wipe extra watercolor off the brush back into the bowl. Rinse the brush in fresh water when switching colors.

3 Toast the bread and top as desired.

4 Throw away leftover watercolors.

PREPARATION TIME
10 minutes

GOOD TO KNOW

You may also use white bread to make the toast.

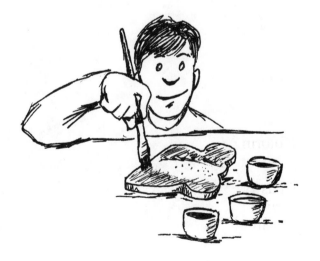

SERVINGS
2

SERVING SIZE
1 slice

Nutrition information for 1 serving

Calories 69
Total fat . . . . 1 g
Saturated fat . . . . 0 g
Cholesterol . . . . 0 mg
Sodium . . . . 148 mg
Total carbohydrate . . . . . 13 g
Fiber . . . . 2 g
Protein . . . . 3 g

Exchanges

1 Starch

Berry Bangle Bracelets

X is for X-tra special projects.

WHAT YOU'LL NEED

- A large dull needle
- Thick thread or fishing line
- Dried fruits and berries such as blueberries, cranberries, raisins, golden raisins, apricots, cherries, or dried apples

WHAT YOU'LL DO

String the fruits and berries on the thread or fishing line to make a bracelet. Tie a secure knot to hold fruit in place.

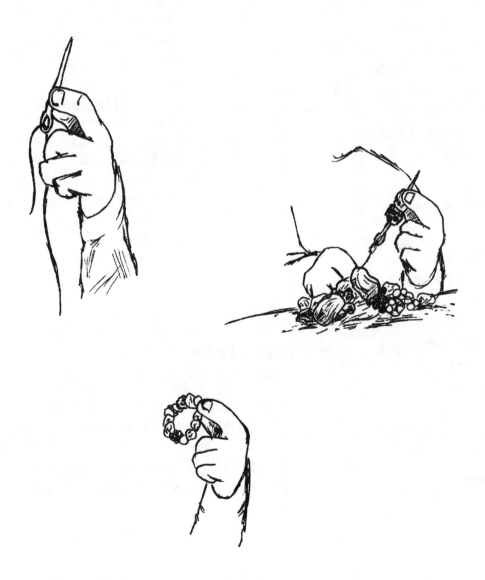

Garlic Cheddar yeast Rolls

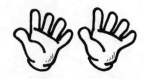

Y is for yeast rolls.

INGREDIENTS

cooking spray

3 tablespoons stick margarine, melted

1 teaspoon garlic powder

1/2 cup + **1** tablespoon (2 1/4 ounces) finely shredded cheddar cheese

1 (11.3-ounce) can quick dinner roll dough

EQUIPMENT

Knife

Cutting board

Grater (optional)

Bowl (or pan; for margarine)

Measuring spoons

Measuring cups

Muffin tin

2 small mixing bowls

Long-handled mixing spoon

Potholders

Foil (optional)

Spoon

DO THIS FIRST

▌ Check with an adult before cooking and ask for help at the oven and with the cutting and grater.

▌ Melt margarine.

▌ If not using prepackaged shredded cheese, grate enough cheddar cheese to make 1/2 cup.

DIRECTIONS

1 Preheat oven to 375°F.

2 Coat a muffin tin with cooking spray and set aside (do not use paper muffin liners).

3 Combine melted margarine and garlic powder in a small bowl, stir well, and set aside.

4 Place cheese in a separate bowl and set aside.

5 The can of roll dough should contain 8 pieces of dough. Cut each piece of dough into 4 equal pieces.

6 Quickly dip each piece of dough in the margarine mixture and then lightly roll in cheese, coating the dough very lightly with cheese.

7 Put 4 pieces of dough in each muffin cup.

8 Bake for 15–19 minutes or until rolls are golden brown on top and done in the centers. If rolls begin to brown too much, lay a sheet of foil over them.

9 Carefully loosen rolls from the muffin tin with a spoon.

PREPARATION TIME
10 minutes

BAKING TIME
15–19 minutes

SERVES
8

SERVING SIZE
1 roll

Nutrition information for 1 serving

Calories	181
Total fat	9 g
Saturated fat	2 g
Cholesterol	8 mg
Sodium	369 mg
Total carbohydrate	18 g
Fiber	1 g
Protein	6 g

Exchanges

1 Starch
2 Fat

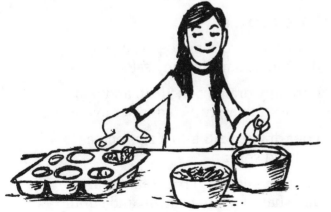

Ziti and Shrimp on a Stick

Z is for ziti.

INGREDIENTS

2 ounces uncooked ziti pasta (about 3/4 cup)

8 ounces frozen, fully-cooked shrimp, thawed

1/4 cup light Caesar salad dressing

EQUIPMENT

Measuring cups

Pan

Strainer

Zip-top bag

8 bamboo skewers (6 inch)

Plate

Plastic wrap

DO THIS FIRST

▌ Check with an adult before you begin cooking and ask for help at the stove.

▌ Read through the whole recipe and make sure you have all of the ingredients and equipment you need.

▌ Thaw shrimp and pat dry.

DIRECTIONS

1 Cook ziti according to package directions, omitting any salt.

2 Carefully drain cooked ziti and pour into a strainer; run cold water over it.

3 Pour drained ziti into a zip-top bag and add shrimp.

4 Pour dressing into bag, seal tightly, and shake well to coat ziti and shrimp with dressing.

5 Refrigerate for at least 6–8 hours to marinate ziti and shrimp.

6 Onto each skewer, thread 1 shrimp, 2 ziti, 1 shrimp, 2 ziti, 1 shrimp, 2 ziti, and 1 shrimp; push skewer through the center of each piece of ziti, not through the hollow opening.

7 Cover and refrigerate until serving time.

PREPARATION TIME **20 minutes**

CHILLING TIME **6–8 hours**

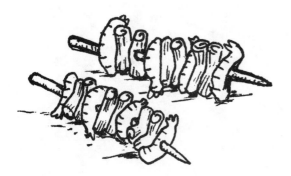

SERVES
8

SERVING SIZE
1 skewer

Nutrition information for 1 serving

Calories	71
Total fat	2 g
Saturated fat	0 g
Cholesterol	55 mg
Sodium	142 mg
Total carbohydrate	6 g
Fiber	0 g
Protein	7 g

Exchanges

1/2 Starch
1 Meat, very lean

Recipe Section 3

. . . .

Last but Not Least

Delicious desserts that are great
after any meal

Rainbow Angel Food Cupcakes

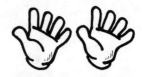

A is for angel food cake.

INGREDIENTS

1 (16-ounce) box angel food cake mix

1 1/4 cups cold water

blue food coloring

yellow food coloring

green food coloring

4 1/2 cups frozen light whipped topping, thawed

EQUIPMENT

Electric mixer

Measuring cups

Muffin pans

33 paper baking cups

3 large mixing bowls

Long-handled mixing spoon

Potholders

Wire rack

DO THIS FIRST

- Check with an adult before you begin cooking and ask for help at the oven and with the electric mixer.

- Read through the whole recipe and make sure you have all of the ingredients and equipment you need.

- Thaw frozen whipped topping.

DIRECTIONS

1 Preheat oven to 350°F.

2 Line muffin pans with 33 paper baking cups; set aside.

3 Place cake mix and water in a large mixing bowl and beat with an electric mixer on low speed for 30 seconds, increase speed to medium and beat 1 minute more.

4 Pour 1/3 of batter into a second bowl and another 1/3 of batter into a third bowl.

5 Carefully stir 9 drops blue food coloring into one bowl of batter, mixing well.

6 Carefully stir 9 drops yellow food coloring into a second bowl of batter, mixing well.

7 Carefully stir 9 drops green food coloring into the third bowl of batter, mixing well.

8 Into each muffin cup, spoon 1 layer of blue batter, then 1 layer of yellow batter, and top with 1 layer of green batter, filling muffin cups 3/4 full.

9 Bake 11 minutes, or until cupcakes begin to turn golden with deep cracks on top.

10 Remove to wire rack and cool completely.

11 Frost cooled cupcakes with light whipped topping right before serving. Refrigerate leftovers.

PREPARATION TIME
25 minutes

BAKING TIME
11 minutes per pan

COOLING TIME
30 minutes

SERVINGS
33

SERVING SIZE
1 cupcake

Nutrition information for 1 serving

Calories	72
Total fat	1 g
Saturated fat	1 g
Cholesterol	0 mg
Sodium	118 mg
Total carbohydrate	14 g
Fiber	0 g
Protein	1 g

Exchanges

1 Starch

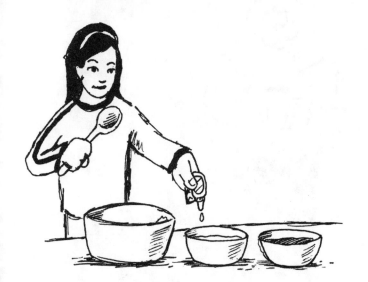

Banana Surprise

B is for banana.

INGREDIENTS

1 medium firm, ripe banana
(about 6 ounces)

2 teaspoons peanut butter chips

1 teaspoon mini semisweet chocolate
chips

1 tablespoon miniature marshmallows

EQUIPMENT

Knife

Cutting board

Measuring spoons

Aluminum foil

Potholders

Spoon

DO THIS FIRST

▌ Check with an adult
before you begin
cooking and ask for
help at the oven and
with cutting.

▌ Read through the
whole recipe and
make sure you have
all of the ingredients
and equipment you
need.

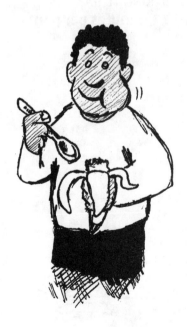

DIRECTIONS

1 Preheat oven to 400°F.

2 Peel back, but do not remove, a 1-inch-wide strip of banana peel. Cut a slit along the length of the banana. Be careful not to cut all the way through the banana.

3 Push the peanut butter chips and chocolate chips down into the slit in the banana, then push in marshmallows.

4 Replace the strip of banana peel. Wrap the banana in aluminum foil.

5 Turn off the oven. Put the banana in the oven for about 10 minutes, or until the marshmallows begin to melt.

6 Eat with a spoon while warm.

PREPARATION TIME
10 minutes

BAKING TIME
10 minutes

SERVES
2

SERVING SIZE
1/2 banana

Nutrition information for 1 serving

Calories 97
Total fat . . . . 2 g
   Saturated fat . . . . 2 g
Cholesterol . . . . 0 mg
Sodium . . . . 13 mg
Total carbohydrate . . . . . 19 g
   Fiber . . . . 2 g
Protein . . . . 2 g

Exchanges

1 Fruit
1/2 Fat

"Souper" Cantaloupe Soup

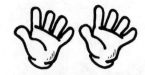

C is for cantaloupe.

INGREDIENTS

1 small banana (about 4 ounces)

4-3/4 cups cantaloupe balls (about 1 medium cantaloupe), divided

1/2 cup green grapes

1 kiwi

1 nectarine (about 5 ounces)

1 plum (about 3 ounces)

1/4 cup unsweetened orange juice concentrate, thawed

1 (8-ounce) container fat-free, artificially-sweetened vanilla-flavored yogurt

1 cup small strawberries with leaves removed

1 1/4 cups rainbow sherbet

DO THIS FIRST

- Check with an adult before you begin cooking and ask for help with cutting and using the blender.

- Read through the whole recipe and make sure you have all of the ingredients and equipment you need.

- Use a melon scoop to make cantaloupe balls, or use a knife to cut cantaloupe into cubes.

- Thaw orange juice concentrate.

- Remove leaves from the strawberries.

EQUIPMENT

Knife

Cutting board

Blender

Melon scoop (optional)

Measuring cups

5 Bowls

DIRECTIONS

1 Slice banana; set aside.

2 Slice grapes in half; set aside.

3 Peel kiwi, cut in half along the length of the kiwi, then cut each half into slices; set aside.

4 Slice nectarine (leaving the skin on); set aside. Throw away the pit.

5 Slice plum (leaving the skin on); set aside. Throw away the pit.

6 Place orange juice concentrate, banana slices, 3 cups of cantaloupe balls, and vanilla yogurt in a blender. Put on blender lid tightly. Blend until smooth.

7 Pour about 1/2 cup of "soup" into each of 5 bowls. Add equal amounts of the remaining cantaloupe balls, sliced grapes, kiwi slices, nectarine slices, plum slices, and strawberries to each bowl. Top with a 1/4 cup scoop of rainbow sherbet.

PREPARATION TIME
25 minutes

SERVINGS
5

SERVING SIZE
1/5 of recipe (about 1 1/2 cups)

**Nutrition information
for 1 serving**

Calories.	238
Total fat.	2 g
Saturated fat	0 g
Cholesterol	3 mg
Sodium	63 mg
Total carbohydrate.	55 g
Fiber	4 g
Protein.	5 g

Exchanges

1 Starch
2 1/2 Fruit

▌ If you don't want to serve all of the "soup" at one time, refrigerate the extra soup before you add fruit or sherbet to it. Store the fruit in air-tight containers in the refrigerator (be sure to toss banana slices, nectarine slices, and plum slices with orange or pineapple juice to keep them from turning brown). Use "soup" and fruit within 2 days.

▌ For smaller appetites, spread "soup," fruit, and sherbet between 10 mugs or small bowls.

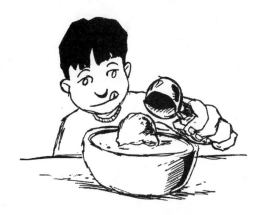

Just Peachy Dumpling Cobbler

D is for dumpling.

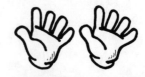

INGREDIENTS

cooking spray

1 (4 1/2-ounce) can biscuits

1 (15-ounce) can spiced peaches in light syrup

water

1/8 teaspoon cinnamon

light whipped topping (optional)

EQUIPMENT

Can opener

Measuring spoons

Knife

Cutting board

2-cup liquid measuring cup

Deep pan with lid

Long-handled mixing spoon

DIRECTIONS

1 Spray a knife with cooking spray. Open biscuits and cut each biscuit into 4 pieces; set aside.

2 Drain syrup off peaches into a 2-cup liquid measuring cup. Add enough water to make 1 1/2 cups liquid; set aside.

3 Cut peaches into bite-sized pieces; set aside.

4 Pour the syrup mixture into a deep pan. Add cinnamon and cover the pan with a lid. Bring to a boil over high heat.

5 Remove lid and use a long-handled spoon to carefully lower 3–4 pieces of dough at a time into the syrup until all the dough is in the pan. Stir to separate dough pieces.

6 Put the lid back on the pan, reduce heat to medium-low, and cook for 4–5 minutes, removing the lid and stirring periodically. The biscuit dough will puff up, then deflate to make dense dumplings when they're fully cooked.

7 Stir in peaches and cover pan.

8 Cook 5 minutes longer, or until the sauce is at desired thickness. The sauce will thicken further upon cooling.

9 Serve with light whipped topping, if desired.

PREPARATION TIME
20 minutes

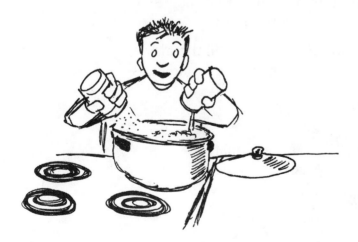

GOOD TO KNOW

If you can't find spiced peaches in your grocery, increase the cinnamon to 1/4 teaspoon and add 1/8 teaspoon nutmeg. Add both spices in step 4.

SERVINGS
5

SERVING SIZE
1/5 of recipe

**Nutrition information
for 1 serving
(without whipped topping):**

Calories	97
Total fat	1 g
Saturated fat	0 g
Cholesterol	0 mg
Sodium	222 mg
Total carbohydrate	21 g
Fiber	1 g
Protein	2 g

Exchanges

1 Starch
1/2 Fruit

Stained Glass Candy Ornaments!

E is for evergreen, like a Christmas tree.

WHAT YOU'LL NEED

Aluminum foil

Cookie sheet

Heavy metal cookie cutters

Cooking spray

2 bags Life Savers candies (will make 10–12 ornaments)

Potholders

Straw

Ribbon

WHAT YOU'LL DO

1 Preheat oven to 350°F.

2 Line cookie sheet with aluminum foil and spray cookie sheet and cutters with nonstick cooking spray.

3 Lay cookie cutters flat on aluminum foil and fill the inside with a single layer of Life Savers, using as many candies as will fit.

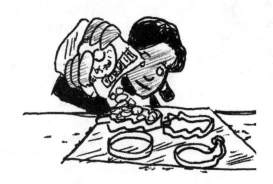

4 Bake 5–7 minutes until candies are melted. Remove from oven and allow candy to cool for about 2 minutes.

5 Make a hole in each ornament with a straw so ribbon can be threaded through for hanging.

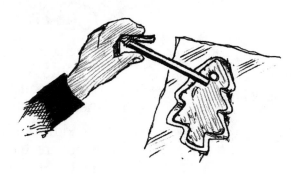

6 Continue cooling until cutters can be handled. Gently pull cutters away from ornament—handle carefully, because the ornaments can break easily!

7 Thread the ornaments with ribbons and hang on your tree or in your windows.

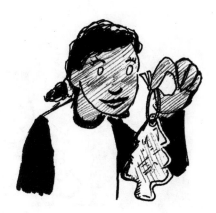

Fun Fruit Kabobs

F is for fruit.

INGREDIENTS

4 small strawberries (or 2 large strawberries sliced in half lengthwise) with green leaves removed

4 banana slices (equal to 1/4 of a small 4-ounce banana)

4 green grapes

4 (2 1/4-inch) pretzel sticks

EQUIPMENT

Knife

Cutting board

DO THIS FIRST

- Check with an adult before you begin cooking and ask for help with slicing.
- Read through the whole recipe and make sure you have all of the ingredients and equipment you need.
- Remove leaves from strawberries.
- Cut 4 banana slices.

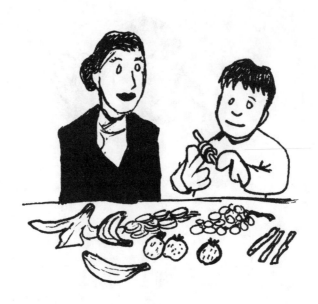

DIRECTIONS

1 Gently push 1 strawberry, 1 banana slice, and 1 grape onto each pretzel stick. Twist pretzel as you are pushing fruit onto it to keep the pretzel from breaking.

2 Eat right away to keep the pretzels crunchy.

PREPARATION TIME
5 minutes

SERVINGS
1

SERVING SIZE
4 fruit kabobs

**Nutrition information
for 1 serving**

Calories	49
Total fat	0 g
Saturated fat:	0 g
Cholesterol	0 mg
Sodium	35 mg
Total carbohydrate	12 g
Fiber	2 g
Protein	1 g

Exchanges

1 Fruit

Graham Crackerwiches

G is for graham cracker.

INGREDIENTS

1 cup fat-free artificially-sweetened vanilla-flavored ice cream

1/2 teaspoon sprinkles, any flavor

8 (2 1/2-inch) graham cracker squares

1 teaspoon chocolate Magic Shell topping

EQUIPMENT

Measuring cups

Measuring spoons

Small cup (or bowl)

Small tray

Ice cream scoop (or big spoon)

Airtight container (optional)

DO THIS FIRST

▎ Check with an adult before you begin cooking.

▎ Read through the whole recipe and make sure you have all of the ingredients and equipment you need.

DIRECTIONS

1 Set ice cream out on the counter for 10–15 minutes to soften.

2 Measure sprinkles into a small cup or bowl; set aside.

3 Lay 4 graham cracker squares on a small tray.

4 Scoop 1/4 cup ice cream on top of each graham cracker square. Carefully spread ice cream to the edges of each graham cracker, taking care not to crack the graham cracker.

5 Top the ice cream with remaining graham crackers to make "sandwiches."

6 Drizzle the top graham cracker of each sandwich with 1/4 teaspoon Magic Shell.

7 Hold graham cracker sandwiches over the sprinkles bowl and lightly sprinkle the sprinkles onto the edges of the ice cream, letting extra sprinkles fall back into the bowl. Lay sandwiches back on the tray.

8 Place the tray in the freezer for 5 minutes, or until the Magic Shell hardens.

9 Serve right away, or store the graham cracker sandwiches in an airtight container in the freezer.

PREPARATION TIME
15 minutes

FREEZING TIME
5 minutes

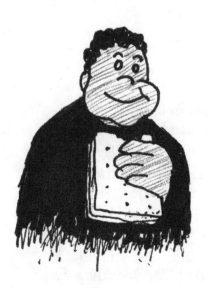

SERVES
4

SERVING SIZE
1 crackerwich

Nutrition information for 1 serving

Calories. 115
Total fat: . . . . .2 g
   Saturated fat . . . . .1 g
Cholesterol. . . . . .0 mg
Sodium: . . . . .111 mg
Total carbohydrate. . . . .21 g
   Fiber . . . . .0 g
Protein. . . . . .3 g

Exchanges

1 1/2 Carbohydrate

Jiggly Honeydew Melon

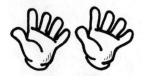

H is for honeydew melon.

INGREDIENTS

1 large honeydew melon, chilled (about 5 pounds)

1 1/2 cups boiling water

2 (0.3-ounce) packages artificially-sweetened strawberry-flavored gelatin

1/2 cup chilled diet strawberry- or raspberry-flavored sparkling water

EQUIPMENT

Knife

Cutting board

Measuring cups

Pan

Spoon

Paper towel

Large bowl

Whisk

DIRECTIONS

1 Slice the melon in half lengthwise. Cut a thin slice from the bottom of each halve so it will stand up.

2 Scoop the seeds out of the melon halves, then turn the melon upside down on a paper towel to drain well.

3 Place boiling water in a large bowl, then whisk in gelatin until it's dissolved. Add chilled sparkling water and whisk until combined.

4 Turn melon halves upright and carefully pour gelatin into them.

5 Carefully place filled melon halves into the refrigerator and chill until firm (about 3 hours).

6 When the gelatin is set, slice each melon halve into 4 wedges.

PREPARATION TIME
15 minutes

CHILLING TIME
3 hours

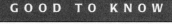

G O O D   T O   K N O W

You can use club soda in place of the sparkling water.

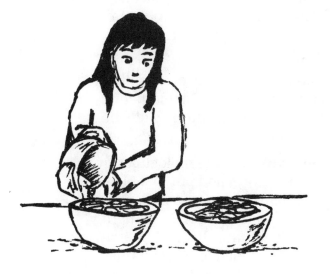

SERVINGS
8

SERVING SIZE
1 slice (1/8 melon)

**Nutrition information
for 1 serving**

Calories	54
Total fat	0 g
Saturated fat	0 g
Cholesterol	0 mg
Sodium	72 mg
Total carbohydrate	13 g
Fiber	1 g
Protein	2 g

Exchanges

1 Fruit

Chocolate-Covered Banana Slushy

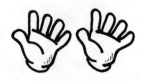

I is for instant beverage.

INGREDIENTS

3 cups fat-free milk, divided

1/4 cup artificially-sweetened chocolate instant beverage mix (such as Nesquik)

1 medium banana (about 6 ounces)

EQUIPMENT

Blender

Measuring cups

Pitcher

Whisk

Ice cube trays

Long-handled mixing spoon

Zip-top freezer bag (optional)

DO THIS FIRST

▎ Check with an adult before you begin cooking and ask for help with the blender.

▎ Read through the whole recipe and make sure you have all of the ingredients and equipment you need.

DIRECTIONS

1 In a pitcher, combine milk and chocolate instant beverage mix. Mix with a whisk until chocolate powder is dissolved.

2 Carefully pour chocolate milk into ice cube trays (about 2 tablespoons per cube) and freeze until solid (about 2 hours).

3 Remove chocolate milk cubes from ice cube trays and put in a blender. Pour remaining 1 cup milk over the cubes, place blender lid on tightly, and blend until slushy. You may need to stop the blender several times, remove the lid, and scrape down the blender or push cubes to the bottom. Remember to put the lid back on before you start the blender again.

4 Add the banana and blend again until slushy.

5 Serve right away.

PREPARATION TIME
15 minutes

FREEZING TIME
2 hours

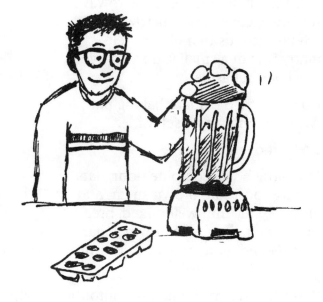

SERVES
8

SERVING SIZE
1/2 cup

**Nutrition information
for 1 serving**

Calories	56
Total fat	0 g
Saturated fat	0 g
Cholesterol	2 mg
Sodium	69 mg
Total carbohydrate	10 g
Fiber	1 g
Protein	4 g

Exchanges

1 Starch

Jolly Jam Bars

J is for jam.

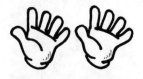

INGREDIENTS

5 tablespoons light stick margarine
  cooking spray
1 cup all-purpose flour
1 cup uncooked quick oats
1/2 teaspoon baking soda
1/8 teaspoon salt
1/2 cup packed light brown sugar
1/4 teaspoon allspice
3/4 cup blackberry 100% fruit spread
1/4 cup powdered sugar
1 teaspoon water

EQUIPMENT

Measuring spoons
Measuring cups
Microwave-safe dish with
  lid (or saucepan)
8″ x 8″ baking pan
Large mixing bowl
Long-handled
  mixing spoon
Potholders
Small bowl
Spoon

DO THIS FIRST

▌Check with an adult before you begin cooking and ask for help at the micro-wave/stove and oven.

▌Read through the whole recipe and make sure you have all of the ingredients and equipment you need.

DIRECTIONS

1 Place the margarine in a microwave-safe dish, cover, and microwave 15–20 seconds to melt, or melt margarine in a small saucepan over low heat; set aside.

2 Coat an 8″ x 8″ square baking pan with cooking spray; set aside.

3 Preheat oven to 350°F.

4 In a large bowl, combine flour, oats, baking soda, salt, brown sugar, and allspice; stir until well mixed, break-ing up any clumps of brown sugar. Add melted margarine and stir until mixture is crumbly.

5 Press 1/2 the crumb mixture into the baking pan, covering the bottom of the pan evenly; set rest aside.

6 Bake 5–7 minutes, or until golden.

7 Spread fruit spread evenly over crust.

8 Sprinkle evenly with remaining crumb mixture.

9 Bake 15–20 minutes, or until topping is golden.

10 Cool completely.

11 In a small bowl, stir together powdered sugar and water to make a glaze. If desired, add 1–2 drops water to make a thinner glaze. Drizzle glaze over bars with a spoon.

12 Allow powdered sugar glaze to dry (about 15–20 minutes), then cut into 16 bars.

PREPARATION TIME
20 minutes

BAKING TIME
20–27 minutes

COOLING TIME
30 minutes

STANDING TIME
15–20 minutes

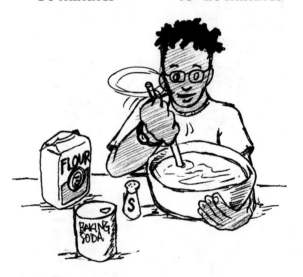

GOOD TO KNOW

You can substitute any flavor of fruit spread in place of blackberry.

SERVES
16

SERVING SIZE
1 bar

Nutrition information for 1 serving

Calories	127
Total fat	2 g
Saturated fat	0 g
Cholesterol	0 mg
Sodium	88 mg
Total carbohydrate	25 g
Fiber	1 g
Protein	2 g

Exchanges

1 1/2 Starch
1/2 Fat

Kiwi-Strawberry "Mock"tail

K is for kiwi.

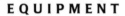

INGREDIENTS

4 kiwis, chilled

1 (10-ounce) package no-sugar-added frozen strawberries, partially thawed

2 (12-ounce) cans diet ginger ale, chilled

EQUIPMENT

Peeler (or paring knife)

Blender

Long-handled mixing spoon

Large pitcher

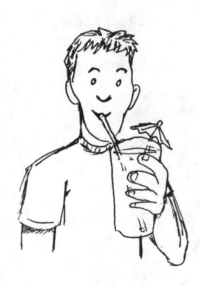

DIRECTIONS

1 Peel kiwis and place in a blender. Put blender lid on tightly and blend kiwis until they are liquid.

2 Add partially thawed strawberries to the blender, put blender lid on tightly, and blend until the fruit makes a thick liquid (there may be a few lumps). Thin with 1/2 can ginger ale if fruit is too thick to blend. If needed, turn off the blender, remove the lid, and push strawberries to the bottom. Remember to put the lid back on before you start the blender again.

3 Pour into a large pitcher and stir in remaining ginger ale until well mixed.

PREPARATION TIME
20 minutes

GOOD TO KNOW

This drink should be served right away or it will lose its fizz.

SERVINGS
11

SERVING SIZE
1/2 cup

Nutrition information for 1 serving

Calories	29
Total fat	0 g
Saturated fat	0 g
Cholesterol	0 mg
Sodium	15 mg
Total carbohydrate	7 g
Fiber	2 g
Protein	0 g

Exchanges

1/2 Fruit

Lemon Ladyfinger Pie

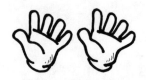

L is for lemon.

INGREDIENTS

2 (0.3-ounce) boxes artificially-sweetened lemon-flavored gelatin

1 1/2 cups boiling water

1/2 cup cold water + ice cubes to make 1 1/4 cups total

1 (3-ounce) package ladyfingers

1 (8-ounce) container fat-free, artificially-sweetened lemon-flavored yogurt

2 cups whole strawberries

EQUIPMENT

Knife

Cutting board

Pan

Measuring cups

2 medium mixing bowls

Long-handled mixing spoon

9-inch deep-dish pie plate

Whisk

DO THIS FIRST

- Check with an adult before you begin cooking and ask for help with cutting and at the stove/microwave.
- Read through the whole recipe and make sure you have all of the ingredients and equipment you need.
- Boil 1 1/2 cups water.

DIRECTIONS

1 Pour gelatin in a bowl and add boiling water. Stir until gelatin is dissolved.

2 Stir in cold water and ice cubes until the ice is nearly melted.

3 Pour 1 1/2 cups gelatin into a separate bowl and refrigerate until thickened, but not totally set (about 45 minutes).

4 Also refrigerate remaining gelatin until slightly thickened (about 25 minutes).

5 When the gelatin from step 3 is ready, cut ladyfingers in half crosswise. Line the bottom and sides of a 9-inch deep-dish pie plate with the ladyfingers and set aside.

6 Whisk yogurt into the slightly thickened gelatin from step 3 until well blended. Pour into pie plate, covering the ladyfingers in the bottom of the pie plate. Push down any ladyfingers that float up; set aside.

7 Remove green leaves and slice strawberries. Arrange sliced strawberries on yogurt layer.

8 Spoon the thickened gelatin from step 2 over the strawberries.

9 Refrigerate again, uncovered, for 2 hours or until firm. Cover and keep refrigerated until serving time.

10 Slice pie into 8 equal servings.

PREPARATION TIME
30 minutes

CHILLING TIME
2 hours 45 minutes

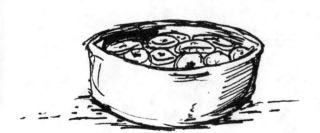

SERVES
8

SERVING SIZE
1/8 pie

Nutrition information for 1 serving

Calories	79
Total fat	1 g
Saturated fat	0 g
Cholesterol	12 mg
Sodium	87 mg
Total carbohydrate	16 g
Fiber	1 g
Protein	3 g

Exchanges

1 Starch

Purple Cow Slushy

M is for milk.

INGREDIENTS

1 (8-ounce) carton fat-free artificially-sweetened vanilla-flavored yogurt

1/2 cup fat-free milk

1 cup frozen unsweetened blueberries, partially thawed

1 1/2 cups ice cubes

EQUIPMENT

Blender

Measuring cups

Glasses

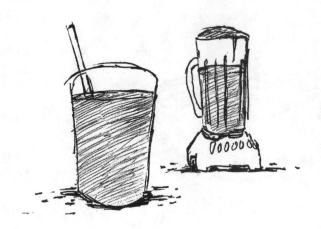

DIRECTIONS

1 Combine yogurt, milk, and 1/2 the blueberries in a blender. Cover tightly and blend.

2 Turn off blender, remove lid, and add remaining blueberries. Cover again and blend until smooth (there may be a few pieces of blueberry skin left).

3 Add ice cubes, cover tightly, and blend until slushy.

4 Pour into glasses and serve right away.

PREPARATION TIME
10 minutes

GOOD TO KNOW

If you want a sweeter-tasting drink, you can add artificial sweetener in step 3.

SERVINGS
4

SERVING SIZE
2/3 cup

**Nutrition information
for 1 serving**

Calories	61
Total fat	0 g
Saturated fat	0 g
Cholesterol	2 mg
Sodium	46 mg
Total carbohydrate	12 g
Fiber	1 g
Protein	3 g

Exchanges

1/2 Fruit
1/2 Milk, fat-free

Nectarine Cups

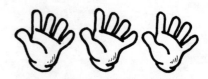

N is for nectarine.

INGREDIENTS

1 tablespoon sugar

1/2 teaspoon cinnamon

4 (6-inch) flour tortillas

butter-flavored cooking spray

1 nectarine

1 (8-ounce) cup fat-free artificially-sweetened vanilla-flavored yogurt

EQUIPMENT

Knife

Cutting board

Measuring spoons

Measuring cups

Small mixing bowl

Paper towels

Spoon

Muffin tin

Potholders

Wire rack

DO THIS FIRST

▌ Check with an adult before you begin cooking and ask for help at the oven, microwave, and with cutting.

▌ Read through the whole recipe and make sure you have all of the ingredients and equipment you need.

DIRECTIONS

1 Preheat oven to 350°F.

2 Combine sugar and cinnamon in a small bowl and mix well; set aside.

3 Place tortillas between 2 damp sheets of paper towel and microwave 30–40 seconds to make them softer and easier to bend.

4 Lightly spray both sides of each tortilla with cooking spray.

5 Use a spoon to lightly sprinkle both sides of each tortilla with the sugar and cinnamon mixture.

6 Hold the edges of each tortilla and squeeze together to form a "cup." Press each tortilla cup into a muffin tin to form a cup with ruffled edges. Press down the center of the tortilla cup to make the bottom of the cup as flat as possible.

7 Bake for 10–12 minutes, or until the tortilla cups are light golden and crisp.

8 Remove tortilla cups from the muffin tin and cool completely on a wire rack.

9 Thinly slice the nectarine; set aside.

10 Spoon 1/4 cup yogurt into each tortilla cup and top with nectarine slices, sticking the ends of the slices down into the yogurt.

11 Serve right away, in small bowls if you wish.

PREPARATION TIME
20 minutes

BAKING TIME
10–12 minutes

COOLING TIME
15 minutes

SERVINGS
4

SERVING SIZE
1 nectarine cup

Nutrition information for 1 serving

Calories	157
Total fat	2 g
Saturated fat	1 g
Cholesterol	1 mg
Sodium	173 mg
Total carbohydrate	30 g
Fiber	2 g
Protein	5 g

Exchanges

1 Starch
1 Fruit
1/2 Milk, fat-free

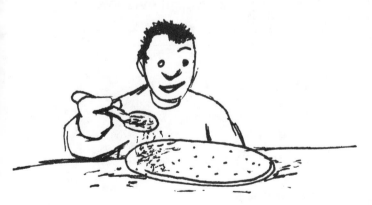

Cinnamon Oat Crunch Topping

O is for oats.

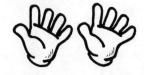

INGREDIENTS

3/4 cup old-fashioned rolled oats, uncooked

1/4 cup oat bran hot cereal, uncooked

1/4 cup wheat germ, lightly toasted

1 1/2 teaspoons cinnamon

2 teaspoons stick margarine, melted

2 tablespoons honey

1 tablespoon packed dark brown sugar

EQUIPMENT

Toaster oven (optional)

Microwave-safe bowl (or small saucepan)

Measuring cups

Measuring spoons

Mixing bowl

Baking sheet

Potholders

DO THIS FIRST

▌ Check with an adult before you begin cooking and ask for help at the oven and stove/microwave.

▌ Read through the whole recipe and make sure you have all of the ingredients and equipment you need.

▌ Lightly toast the wheat germ in the oven or toaster oven.

▌ Melt 2 teaspoons margarine in the microwave for 15–20 seconds or on the stove in a small saucepan over low heat.

DIRECTIONS

1 Preheat oven to 350°F.

2 Combine all of the ingredients in a bowl and mix until moistened.

3 Spread on an ungreased baking sheet and bake for 8–10 minutes, or until dry. Watch closely during the last 2 minutes and remove from the oven, if needed, to prevent over-browning.

4 Cool completely.

PREPARATION TIME
10 minutes

BAKING TIME
8–10 minutes

COOLING TIME
30 minutes

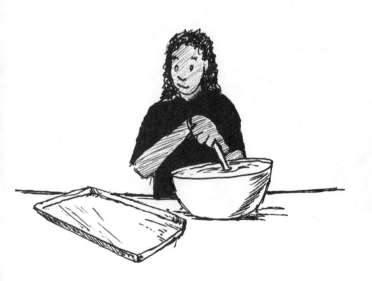

SERVINGS
7

SERVING SIZE
1/4 cup

Nutrition information for 1 serving

Calories	102
Total fat	3 g
Saturated fat	1 g
Cholesterol	0 mg
Sodium	14 mg
Total carbohydrate	18 g
Fiber	3 g
Protein	3 g

Exchanges

1 Starch
1/2 Fat

Potato Stampers!

P is for potato.

WHAT YOU'LL NEED

Small red or white potato

Paring knife

Marking pen

Stamp pad

Zip-top bags

WHAT YOU'LL DO

1 Carefully cut the potato in half.

2 With a marking pen, draw your stamp design on the flat part of the cut potato.

3 You can make designs such as smiley faces or someone's initials. Remember to put any letters or words in reverse.

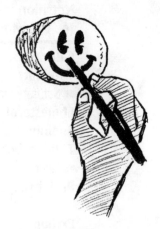

4 Scrape away all of the potato except the area of your drawing.

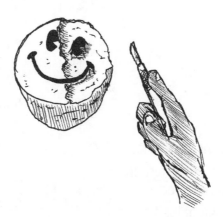

5 Press the potato down on a stamp pad. Stamp your design on papers, notes, or wrapping paper.

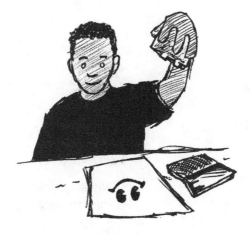

6 Store the potato stampers in zip-top bags in the refrigerator.

Banana-Orange Quick Bread

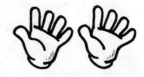

Q is for quick bread.

INGREDIENTS

cooking spray

2 eggs

1 cup well-mashed ripe banana (about 1 1/2 10-inch bananas)

1 (6-ounce) can unsweetened orange juice concentrate, thawed

2 teaspoons pumpkin pie spice

1 teaspoon baking powder

1 teaspoon baking soda

1 1/2 cups flour

1/2 cup quick oats

1/2 cup raisins

EQUIPMENT

Fork (for mashing)

Measuring cups

Measuring spoons

8" loaf pan

Large mixing bowl

Whisk

Long-handled mixing spoon

Toothpick

Potholders

Dull knife

Wire rack

DO THIS FIRST

▌ Check with an adult before you begin cooking and ask for help at the oven.

▌ Read through the whole recipe and make sure you have all of the ingredients and equipment you need.

▌ Mash enough bananas to make 1 cup.

▌ Thaw orange juice concentrate.

DIRECTIONS

1 Preheat oven to 350°F.

2 Coat an 8-inch loaf pan well with cooking spray and set aside.

3 Break eggs into a large mixing bowl. Mix the eggs until frothy, using a wire whisk.

4 Add mashed banana, orange juice concentrate, pumpkin pie spice, baking powder, and baking soda; stir until well mixed.

5 Add flour and oats; stir until just moistened.

6 Stir in raisins.

7 Pour batter into the loaf pan and bake for 45–50 minutes, or until the bread has browned on top and a toothpick inserted into the center of the loaf comes out clean.

8 If needed, loosen sides of the loaf of bread from the pan with a dull knife or metal spatula. Turn bread out on a wire rack to cool.

PREPARATION TIME
15 minutes

BAKING TIME
45-50 minutes

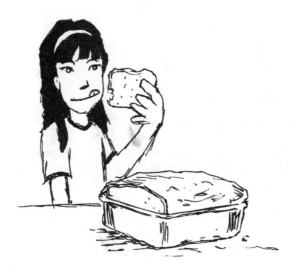

SERVINGS
16

SERVING SIZE
1/2 a 1-inch-thick slice

Nutrition information for 1 serving

Calories. 110
Total fat. . . . . 1 g
 Saturated fat . . . . 0 g
Cholesterol. . . . . 27 mg
Sodium . . . . 111 mg
Total carbohydrate. . . . . 23 g
 Fiber . . . . 1 g
Protein. . . . . 3 g

Exchanges

1 Starch
1/2 Fruit

Mini Pumpkin Raisin Muffins

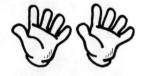

R is for raisin.

INGREDIENTS

cooking spray

6 tablespoons stick margarine

1 cup all-purpose flour

1/4 cup sugar

1 teaspoon baking powder

pinch of salt

1 teaspoon pumpkin pie spice

3/4 cup fat-free milk

1 large egg

1 teaspoon vanilla extract

2 tablespoons artificially-sweetened maple-flavored syrup

1 cup canned pumpkin

1/3 cup raisins

EQUIPMENT

Can opener

Measuring spoons

Measuring cups

Mini-muffin tin

36 paper baking cups

Microwave-safe bowl (or saucepan)

2 large mixing bowls

Whisk

Spoon

Toothpick

Potholders

DO THIS FIRST

▌ Check with an adult before you begin cooking and ask for help with the can opener and at the oven and stove/microwave.

▌ Read through the whole recipe and make sure you have all of the ingredients and equipment you need.

DIRECTIONS

1 Preheat the oven to 400°F.

2 Line mini-muffin tins with 36 paper baking cups. Spray cups with cooking spray, and set aside.

3 Melt the margarine in the microwave for 20–30 seconds, or in a small saucepan over low heat; set aside.

4 In a large bowl, sift together the flour, sugar, baking powder, salt, and pumpkin pie spice; set aside.

5 In a separate bowl, whisk together the melted margarine, milk, egg, vanilla extract, syrup, and pumpkin. Add to the flour mixture and stir until well mixed.

6 Stir in raisins.

7 Spoon batter into mini-muffin cups, filling each one 3/4 full.

8 Bake 21–23 minutes, or until muffins begin to brown on top and a toothpick inserted in the center comes out clean.

PREPARATION TIME
20 minutes

BAKING TIME
21–23 minutes

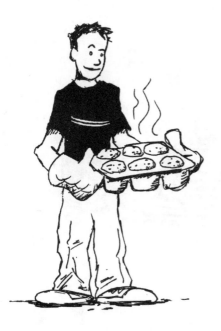

SERVES
18

SERVING SIZE
2 muffins

Nutrition information for 1 serving

Calories	92
Total fat	4 g
Saturated fat	1 g
Cholesterol	12 mg
Sodium	76 mg
Total carbohydrate	12 g
Fiber	1 g
Protein	2 g

Exchanges

1 Starch
1/2 Fat

Towering waffle Sundae

S is for sundae.

INGREDIENTS

3 frozen mini waffles (such as Kellogg's Eggo Minis)

3 tablespoons reduced-fat artificially-sweetened Neapolitan ice cream

2 teaspoons artificially-sweetened chocolate-flavored syrup

1 tablespoon fat-free canned whipped cream

EQUIPMENT

Toaster

Measuring spoons

Bowl (or plate)

Spoon

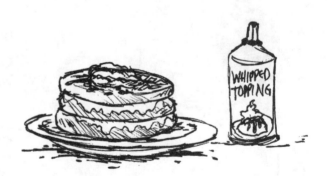

DIRECTIONS

1 Heat waffles in toaster until golden and crisp. Let waffles cool a couple of minutes.

2 Place 1 waffle in a bowl or on a plate and top with 1 tablespoon chocolate ice cream.

3 Stack on a second waffle, then add 1 tablespoon vanilla ice cream.

4 Add the third waffle, then add 1 tablespoon strawberry ice cream.

5 Spray whipped cream on top.

6 Drizzle with chocolate syrup.

PREPARATION TIME
10 minutes

SERVES
1

SERVING SIZE
1 waffle

**Nutrition information
for 1 serving**

Calories	90
Total fat	2 g
Saturated fat	0 g
Cholesterol	4 mg
Sodium	123 mg
Total carbohydrate	15 g
Fiber	0 g
Protein	2 g

Exchanges

1 Starch

Simple Strawberry Tart

T is for tart.

INGREDIENTS

1/3 cup sliced fresh strawberries
artificial sweetener (optional)

1 single-serving (approximately
2/3 ounce) graham cracker crust

1 teaspoon artificially-sweetened
chocolate-flavored syrup

EQUIPMENT

Knife

Cutting board

Measuring cups

Measuring spoons

Small bowl (optional)

Spoon

DO THIS FIRST

▌ Check with an adult
before you begin
cooking and ask for
help with slicing.

▌ Read through the
whole recipe and
make sure you have
all of the ingredients
and equipment you
need.

▌ Slice enough straw-
berries to make
1/3 cup.

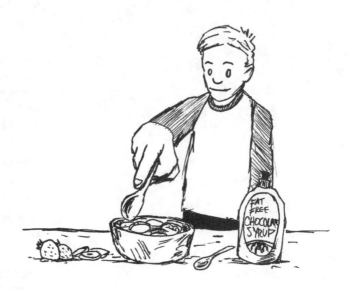

DIRECTIONS

1 If you want sweeter strawberries, place them in a small bowl, sprinkle with artificial sweetener, and stir them well with a spoon.

2 Spoon strawberries into graham cracker crust.

3 Drizzle chocolate-flavored syrup over the berries.

PREPARATION TIME
5 minutes

Serve right away to keep the crust from getting soggy.

SERVINGS
1

SERVING SIZE
1 tart

**Nutrition information
for 1 serving**

Calories	137
Total fat	6 g
Saturated fat	1 g
Cholesterol	0 mg
Sodium	147 mg
Total carbohydrate	19 g
Fiber	2 g
Protein	1 g

Exchanges

1 Starch
1 Fat

Pineapple Upside-Down Cupcakes

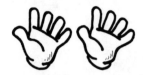

U is for upside-down cake.

INGREDIENTS

- butter-flavored cooking spray
- 1 (8-ounce) box low-fat artificially-sweetened yellow snack cake mix (such as Sweet 'n Low yellow snack cake mix)
- 1 (6-ounce) can unsweetened pineapple juice
- 1/4 teaspoon cinnamon
- 1 tablespoon + 2 teaspoons packed brown sugar
- 10 maraschino cherries, well drained
- 1 (8-ounce) can crushed pineapple in juice, well drained

EQUIPMENT

Electric mixer
Can opener
Sieve
Spoon
Paper towels
Measuring spoons
Muffin tins
10 foil-covered baking cups
Mixing bowls
Long-handled mixing spoon
Spoon
Toothpick
Potholders
Wire rack
Airtight container (optional)

DO THIS FIRST

- Check with an adult before you begin cooking and ask for help at the oven and with the electric mixer and can opener.

- Read through the whole recipe and make sure you have all of the ingredients and equipment you need.

- Open the can of crushed pineapple, pour the pineapple into a sieve, and drain well, forcing the juice out of the pineapple by pressing on it with the back of a spoon.

- Rinse the maraschino cherries and lay them on a paper towel to drain well.

DIRECTIONS

1 Preheat oven to 375°F.

2 Line a muffin tin with 10 foil-covered baking cups. Spray the inside of the baking cups with cooking spray; set aside.

3 Make cake batter according to the package directions, using pineapple juice in place of water; set aside.

4 Sprinkle the bottom of each baking cup lightly and evenly with cinnamon and with 1/2 teaspoon brown sugar. Set a maraschino cherry in the center of each baking cup and sprinkle crushed pineapple around the cherry. Gently press pineapple down with your fingertips.

5 Using a spoon, fill the baking cups nearly full with cake batter.

6 Bake for 20 minutes, or until a toothpick inserted into the center of the cupcakes comes out clean. Take cupcakes from the oven and carefully remove them from the tins to a wire rack. Cool at least 10 minutes.

7 Turn the cupcakes upside down, peel off the paper liner, and eat.

PREPARATION TIME
25 minutes

BAKING TIME
20 minutes

COOLING TIME
10 minutes

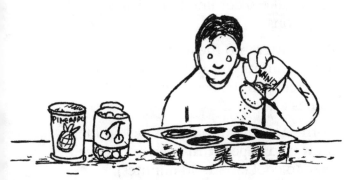

GOOD TO KNOW

Store leftover cupcakes in an airtight container and they will stay fresh for 3–4 days.

SERVES
10

SERVING SIZE
1 cupcake

Nutrition information for 1 serving

Calories	119
Total fat	2 g
Saturated fat	1 g
Cholesterol	0 mg
Sodium	16 mg
Total carbohydrate	27 g
Fiber	1 g
Protein	2 g

Exchanges

2 Starch

Vanilla Polka-Dot Cake

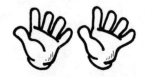

V is for vanilla.

INGREDIENTS

cooking spray

1 (8-ounce) box low-fat artificially-sweetened white snack cake mix (such as Sweet 'n Low white snack cake mix)

1 (1-ounce) package fat-free artificially-sweetened vanilla-flavored instant pudding mix

1 (1.3-ounce) envelope whipped topping mix

1 1/2 cups fat-free milk

2 tablespoons candy-coated milk chocolate candies (such as M&Ms)

EQUIPMENT

Electric mixer

Knife

Cutting board

Measuring cups

Measuring spoons

8" loaf pan

Waxed paper

Mixing bowls

Long-handled mixing spoon

Toothpick

Potholders

Wire rack

Rubber spatula

Plastic wrap

DIRECTIONS

1 Preheat oven to 375°F.

2 Line the bottom only of an 8-inch loaf pan with waxed paper. Coat the sides of the pan with cooking spray. Set pan aside.

3 Make cake according to package directions.

4 Pour batter into the loaf pan and bake for 40 minutes, or until a toothpick inserted into the center of the cake comes out clean.

5 Turn cake out onto a wire rack, pull off waxed paper, turn over, and leave cake to cool (about 30 minutes).

6 In a large bowl, combine pudding mix and whipped topping mix. Add milk and beat at low speed with an electric mixer until blended. Then beat at high speed 4 minutes or until soft peaks form.

7 Slice the cake in half horizontally to make 2 layers. Spread the bottom half with a thick layer of frosting. Carefully set the top half of the cake onto the frosting and frost the outside of the cake with the remaining frosting. Cover and refrigerate cake until serving time.

8 Right before serving, press the candy-coated milk chocolate candies on the top and sides of the cake to make polka-dots.

PREPARATION TIME
20 minutes

BAKING TIME
40 minutes

COOKING TIME
30 minutes

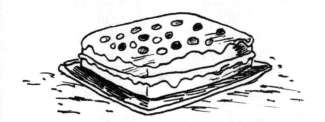

SERVINGS
8

SERVING SIZE
1 (1-inch-thick) slice

Nutrition information for 1 serving

Calories 162
Total fat . . . . 3 g
   Saturated fat . . . . 1 g
Cholesterol . . . . 1 mg
Sodium . . . . 211 mg
Total carbohydrate . . . . . 34 g
   Fiber . . . . 1 g
Protein . . . . 4 g

Exchanges

2 Starch
1/2 Fat

Watermelon Freeze

W is for watermelon.

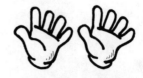

INGREDIENTS

7 cups 1-inch watermelon cubes with seeds removed (about 1/4 a medium watermelon)

1/2 cup frozen unsweetened white grape juice concentrate

2 tablespoons fresh lime juice

EQUIPMENT

Knife

Cutting board

Blender

Measuring cups

Measuring spoons

Baking sheet

Zip-top freezer bag (optional)

Ice cream scoop
  (or big spoon)

DO THIS FIRST

▮ Check with an adult before you begin cooking and ask for help with cutting and the blender.

▮ Read through the whole recipe and make sure you have all of the ingredients and equipment you need.

▮ Cut enough 1-inch watermelon cubes to make 7 cups. Be sure to take out any seeds.

DIRECTIONS

1 Place watermelon chunks in a single layer on a baking sheet. Freeze at least 1 hour, or until very firm (frozen watermelon may be stored in the freezer in a zip-top freezer bag for up to 1 month).

2 Remove watermelon from freezer and let stand at room temperature for 15–20 minutes so that it softens slightly.

3 Place 1/4 of the frozen watermelon plus all of the juice concentrate and lime juice in a blender. Put lid on and. blend until smooth; periodically turn blender off, remove lid, and push watermelon chunks to the bottom with a spoon. Remember to put the lid back on before you start the blender again.

4 Continue blending, adding remaining watermelon a few pieces at a time. Remember to turn the blender off before removing the lid and to put the lid back on before starting the blender again.

5 Freeze any left-over fruit. When ready to serve, let watermelon freeze stand at room temperature for 10 minutes to soften before scooping it into bowls.

PREPARATION TIME
25 minutes

FREEZING TIME
1 hour

STANDING TIME
15–20 minutes

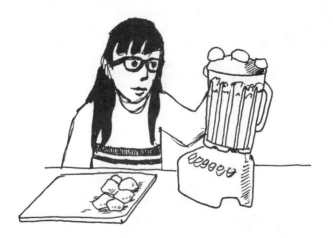

SERVINGS
8

SERVING SIZE
1/2 cup

**Nutrition information
for 1 serving**

Calories	86
Total fat	1 g
Saturated fat	0 g
Cholesterol:	0 mg
Sodium	8 mg
Total carbohydrate	20 g
Fiber	1 g
Protein	1 g

Exchanges

1 1/2 Fruit

Sugar-Free Finger Paint

X is for X-tra special projects.

WHAT YOU'LL NEED

Finger paint paper or butcher paper

Spray bottle filled with water

Small box of artificially-sweetened fruit-flavored gelatin

Paintbrushes

WHAT YOU'LL DO

1 Tape the paper to a table.

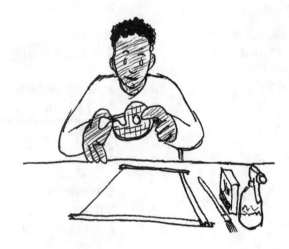

2 Spray water onto the paper and sprinkle the paper with dry gelatin.

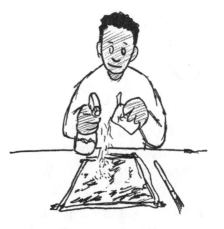

3 Use a brush to "paint" a picture.

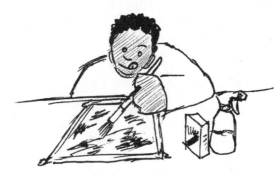

4 As the paper absorbs the gelatin, spray with more water to continue the fun.

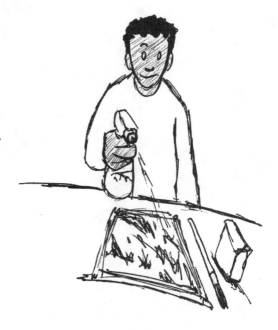

Stained Glass Yogurt

Y is for yogurt.

INGREDIENTS

1 (8-ounce) cup fat-free, artificially-sweetened vanilla-flavored yogurt

1/8 teaspoon dry artificially-sweetened lime-flavored gelatin powder

1/8 teaspoon dry artificially-sweetened strawberry-flavored gelatin powder

EQUIPMENT

Measuring cups
Measuring spoons
Bowl

DO THIS FIRST

▌ Check with an adult before you begin cooking.

▌ Read through the whole recipe and make sure you have all of the ingredients and equipment you need.

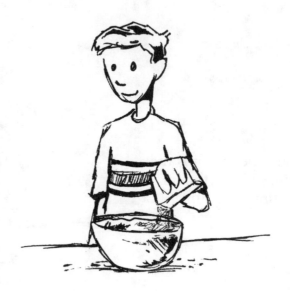

DIRECTIONS

1 Spoon yogurt into a bowl.

2 Sprinkle a design on the yogurt with the lime gelatin powder, then with the strawberry gelatin powder.

3 Let yogurt stand 1–2 minutes until the gelatin powders turn bright green and red.

4 Eat right away.

PREPARATION TIME
5 minutes

SERVES
1

SERVING SIZE
1 cup

**Nutrition information
for 1 serving**

Calories	126
Total fat	0 g
Saturated fat	0 g
Cholesterol	4 mg
Sodium	136 mg
Total carbohydrate	23 g
Fiber	0 g
Protein	8 g

Exchanges

1 1/2 Milk, fat-free

Zoo-rific Zoo Animal Cookie Treats

Z is for zoo animal cookie.

INGREDIENTS

1 (1.4-ounce) box fat-free artificially-sweetened chocolate pudding mix

2 cups fat-free milk

32 zoo animal cookies

EQUIPMENT

Measuring cups

Mixing bowls

Long-handled mixing spoon

Spoon

Airtight container

DIRECTIONS

1 Prepare pudding according to package directions. You'll use about 1/4 cup pudding in this recipe—refrigerate the rest.

2 Lay cookies on the counter with the flat side up.

3 Spoon 1 dollop (about 3/4 teaspoon) pudding on each.

4 Top each with a second cookie with the animal side facing you (you can use 2 of the same animal cookies for each treat) and place in an airtight container.

5 Put lid tightly on the container and carefully place in the freezer. Freeze until pudding is solid (about 1 hour).

6 Remove treats from freezer and let stand at room temperature to soften for about 7–10 minutes before serving.

PREPARATION TIME
10 minutes

FREEZING TIME
1 hour

STANDING TIME
7–10 minutes

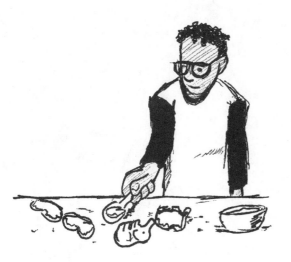

SERVES
4

SERVING SIZE
4 treats

Nutrition information for 1 serving

Calories	99
Total fat	3 g
Saturated fat	1 g
Cholesterol	0 mg
Sodium	101 mg
Total carbohydrate	17 g
Fiber	0 g
Protein	2 g

Exchanges

1 Starch
1/2 Fat

Index
Alphabetical List of Recipes

Subject Index